Reprogramming Pain

Transform Pain and Suffering
Into Health and Success

Developments in Clinical Psychology

Glenn R. Caddy, series editor
Nova University

MMPI-168 Codebook, by Ken R. Vincent, Iliana Castillo, Robert I. Hauser, H. James Stuart, Javier A. Zapata, Cal K. Cohn, and Gregory O'Shanick, 1984

Integrated Clinical and Fiscal Management in Mental Health: A Guidebook, by Fred Newman and James Sorensen, 1986

The Professional Practice of Psychology, edited by Georgiana Shick Tryon, 1986

Clinical Applications of Hypnosis, edited by Frank A. DePiano and Herman C. Salzberg,1986

Full Battery Codebook, by Ken R. Vincent, 1987

Development in the Assessment and Treatment of Addictive Behaviors, edited by Ted D. Nirenberg, 1987

Feminist Psychotherapies, edited by Mary Ann Douglas and Lenore E. Walker, 1988

Child Multimodal Therapy, by Donald B, Keat II, 1990

Psychophysiology for Clinical Psychologists, by Walter W. Surwillo, 1990

Strategic Health Planning: Methods and Techniques Applied to Marketing and Management, by Allen D. Spiegel and Herbert H. Hyman, 1991

Behavioral Medicine: International Perspectives (Vol. 1-3), edited by D.G. Byrne and Glenn R. Caddy, 1992

The MMPI: A Contemporary Normative Study of Adolescents, edited by Robert C. Colligan and Kenneth P. Offord, 1992

Adult-Child Research and Experience, by Robert E. Haskell, 1993

Reprogramming Pain, by Barry Bittman, 1995

Reprogramming Pain

Transform Pain and Suffering
Into Health and Success

Barry Bittman, M.D.

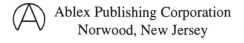

Ablex Publishing Corporation
Norwood, New Jersey

Printed in the United States of America

Bittman, Barry B.
    Reprogramming pain : transform pain and suffering into health and
success / Barry B. Bittman.
        p.   cm. -- (Developments in clinical psychology)
    Includes bibliographical references and index.
    ISBN 1-56750-207-5 (cloth). -- ISBN 1-56750-208-3 (paper : alk.
paper)
    1. Chronic pain--Psychological aspects.   I. Title. II. Series.
RB127.B55   1995
616'.0472--dc20   95-42990
                                                                   CIP

Ablex Publishing Corporation
355 Chestnut Street
Norwood, New Jersey 07648

dedicated to
my wife, Karen
and my children
Benjamin, Marcus and Lauren.

Table of Contents

Foreword   ix

Preface   xi

Acknowledgements   xiii

Chapter 1   The Sacred Alliance   1
             The Relationship Between Mind and Body

Chapter 2   The Origins of Pain   21
             The Brain-Body Circuit

Chapter 3   The Mind's Role   37
             The Invisible Navigator

Chapter 4   The Body's Role   55
             Programming by Movement

Chapter 5   Modern Conditioning   75
             Programming by the Media

Chapter 6   Crossing The Line   93
             Personal Reflections

Chapter 7   Mind/Body   121
             Technology 101
             The Owner's Manual

Chapter 8   Convergent Therapy   143
             Synergy in Pain Care

Chapter 9   The Potential Within   165
             Taking Action

Chapter 10   Reprogramming Pain   185
             10 Logical Steps

Foreword

Reprogramming Pain, by Barry Bittman, M.D., is an important addition for pain patients, physicians, and other clinicians interested in state-of-the-art pain management. Chronic pain is an epidemic. The cost in terms of dollars spent on health care, loss of work, and suffering experienced by patients and their families is staggering. All too often the person in pain is treated as a pariah. Treatment options have been limited to medication and surgery without realistic consideration of alternative approaches. The patient who is seen for five minutes by a doctor and receives no patient education is left to his/her own interpretation of their experience. Is it little wonder that many individuals experiencing pain become anxious, angry or depressed? Unresolved, such pain and suffering becomes a vicious cycle.

Reprogramming Pain explores why this occurs and describes methods for both prevention and intervention. Dr. Bittman helps the reader understand the relation between mind and body and how stress, secondary to unremitting pain, can lead to a hopeless-helpless despair. Written in easy to understand prose, *Reprogramming Pain* educates the reader regarding anatomy, physiology and the role of the mind in the interpretation of painful stimuli. Case stories help heighten awareness of the author's points.

Perhaps the greatest contributions found in *Reprogramming Pain* are the chapters describing the role of learned responses to pain. As Dr. Bittman ably points out, that which is learned can also be reprogrammed. This book is about transferring power from the expert to the ultimate user--the individual experiencing pain. *Reprogramming Pain* encourages the person in pain to take action which can help reduce the intensity, frequency, and duration of pain. Dr. Bittman helps patients assess their situation, work with members of the health care team and establish realistic goals.

Richard S. Weiner, PhD
Executive Director
American Academy of Pain Management

Preface

Chronic pain destroys the quality of life for millions of sufferers in our society. Unfortunately, many of us are programmed to maintain sickness rather than health. Frequently, after a seemingly minor or insignificant injury, a cloak of pain falls upon a victim and suffocates an entire existence. Longstanding pain is more than just hurting. It is a vicious cycle which continuously feeds upon and perpetuates itself. Ongoing pain envelops ones soul, severing meaningful relationships with co-workers, friends and loved ones.

Health care professionals are often frustrated when dealing with the chronic pain sufferer. Most practitioners do not treat the entire person, as this is often overwhelming. It is not surprising that chronic pain is so poorly understood.

The sequence of events leading to a life of chronic pain is often predictable. Pain behavior, to a large extent, is the product of programming by sources that vary from major industries to health care professionals. Physicians and patients alike are encouraged to choose drug after drug for the instant cure. A poor response to the latest weapon in the arsenal of modern medication is unfortunately suggestive of personal failure. As a result, we are severely affected by condescending looks and statements from those who are entrusted with our lives. We place ourselves in the hands of a health care system that is based upon cost effectiveness, with little regard for personal suffering.

Day after day, hundreds or even thousands of times per year, we are programmed by the media to dress, act, appear, deal with pain or even drown our suffering in a manner that is not conducive to our well-being. Through advertising schemes, we are programmed to strike back at pain with a pill. Yet we are surprised and troubled when this action leads to overt addiction.

According to C. David Tollison, Ph.D and editor of the *Handbook of Chronic Pain Management*, approximately 40 million Americans live with chronic pain, accounting for nearly 93 million lost work days each year. The estimated total cost of chronic pain and its treatment is nearly $60 billion annually!

Why does this occur? Can it be prevented? Can we learn to recognize our own programmed pain responses? Can we find health care providers who truly understand suffering and consistently utilize non-pharmacological tools? Can we reprogram ourselves in a manner that promotes good health? The answer to all of these questions is yes. We must learn to focus on ...

REPROGRAMMING PAIN

Acknowledgments

To all of my patients, perhaps my greatest teachers, I extend gratitude for sharing your lives with me. This book would not be possible without your precious lessons.

I am also thankful for the opportunity of working with a wonderful staff, observing and absorbing your insights throughout the years.

Special thanks is extended to Al Losch, Jr. for having the patience to organize the layout of this book.

I am truly indebted to the wonderful friends, scientists and authors who have inspired me to search for new solutions and to believe in the power of the human spirit. You have courageously extended yourselves into new and remarkable realms. Without you, this world would be an empty place.

To Mitchell Ghen, thank you for showing me the Light.

To Karen, my wife, there are no words to express my appreciation for your countless hours reviewing and editing what started out as a mere dream. My work is truly ours. Without you, there would be no more than dreams.

Chapter 1

The Sacred Alliance

The Relationship Between Mind and Body

Which comes first, pain or stress? The answer is often elusive. Thus, the necessity of treating mind and body simultaneously becomes apparent.

This is not just another book about pain. It is about people; ordinary people like you and me and why we develop and live with ongoing pain. *Reprogramming Pain* begins with a practical look at how a seemingly minor injury can become transformed into a lifetime of suffering. This book focuses on the inseparable nature of mind and body on many levels. It explores health care, its providers and the patient-physician relationship. An understanding of the potential impact of this less than perfect system on the chronic pain sufferer is presented.

Through a series of examples and case studies, the following chapters set the stage for understanding how the pain

1

sufferer is programmed in our society. *Reprogramming Pain* is ultimately about hopes, aspirations and relationships. It provides the foundation for learning to reprogram ourselves to live happier and fuller lives.

Reprogramming Pain specifically addresses two fundamental issues. The first focuses on why a potentially serious injury is literally brushed off by certain individuals who enjoy rapid and complete recovery against all odds, while for others, even a seemingly minor event sets the stage for a lifetime of suffering. The second issue explores the question of why accepted medical approaches fail to reestablish normalcy in the lives of chronic pain victims. *Reprogramming Pain* builds on these insights to provide a comprehensive step by step plan to turn failure into success and suffering into health and happiness.

The key to *Reprogramming Pain* is *synergy*. This term refers to the fact that the combined effect of two or more therapeutic strategies performed simultaneously is greater than the total sum of the individual approaches. In essence, one plus one plus one equals more than three when the pain sufferer plays an active role in a synergistic program! The following case history illustrates this concept.

Deborah's Story

A lawyer at a Manhattan law firm, Deborah is a 44-year-old executive, who enjoys tennis and modern dance. During a warm up session one evening at a New York studio, she suddenly noted a harsh cracking sound in her left knee coupled with excruciating, fiery pain that took her breath

2

away. In agony, she was assisted to the bench where ice was applied and the leg was elevated. At a nearby Emergency Room, an orthopedic surgeon ordered x-rays and told her that a cartilaginous structure within the knee had been torn and that arthro-scopic surgery was necessary.

Two days later, the operation proceeded without complications and she was released the following morning. Ongoing pain ensued, while swelling and discoloration was prominent. Unable to commute into the city, Deborah rested at home, alone in New Jersey. By week three, the swelling had resolved and she managed to get a ride to the office. Work, however, piled up despite a team of understanding and sympathetic coworkers and associates.

A follow-up visit with the surgeon disclosed normal, routine healing and physical therapy was prescribed. Unfortunately, after only two treatments limited to hot packs and range of motion exercises, the pain escalated. Therapy was abruptly discontinued and replaced with a prescription for a controlled pain medication. Progressively more despondent, Deborah failed to resume her typical schedule and her law practice suffered. Her air of confidence and control was replaced by doubt and fear.

A consultation with an anaesthesiologist was ordered, yet despite repeated steroid injections into the knee, resolution of pain was not in sight. To worsen matters, hip pain developed due to poor knee stability. Additional pain medications and muscle relaxants were prescribed. As a result, altered sleep patterns translated into overwhelming fatigue that worsened matters considerably.

A sense of remorse and resignation prompted a series of visits to a psychologist. Overt depression was initially diagnosed, yet despite counseling, Deborah continued to be overwhelmed by pain. Job performance suffered and her law firm suggested an extended leave of absence. A lifelong friend and senior member of her firm recommended a consultation with a comprehensive pain and rehabilitation center 20 miles from her home.

The director of the clinic performed a detailed examination and spent approximately one hour outlining what he described as a multidisciplinary treatment approach. He proposed that her dedicated participation in a collaborative treatment program incorporating medical, physical and behavioral approaches simultaneously was the key to resuming a wonderful and pain free existence. Deborah was hesitant to proceed, in view of her recent failures with what appeared to be the very same strategies. The doctor carefully explained that his program was synergistic, implying that the effect of the whole is equal to more than the mere sum of the parts. Her role in reestablishing health was clearly emphasized. He proceeded to explain that physical therapy is best tolerated when performed simultaneously with pain management strategies and that behavioral approaches work best when combined with effective pain reduction modalities.

Within six weeks, Deborah returned to work with new insights about life, herself and her path to a pain free state. Shortly thereafter, she resumed dance classes two evenings a week and two months later, doubles tennis was better than ever.

Deborah's story illustrates the synergistic approach that serves as the basis for *Reprogramming Pain*. Many chronic pain sufferers travel from physician to physician, to psychologist, to chiropractor, to physical therapist without ever experiencing lasting relief. It may not be immediately obvious to the chronic pain sufferer that the best strategy for living free of pain is a synergistic mind/body approach that enlists the subject's active participation.

Deborah did not tolerate physical therapy due to increasing pain, even with passive movement. Injections did not help and were perceived as extremely painful. Psychological intervention was unfocused due to the distraction from constant pain. For the chronic pain sufferer, independent therapeutic approaches often lead to failure.

The mind/body approach finally succeeded for Deborah when appropriate strategies were enlisted synergistically with her active participation. The medical approach enhanced the physical one, which in turn facilitated the behavioral approach. In fact, each intervention when performed in a coordinated, multidisciplinary manner supported the others.

I typically discuss this synergistic effect with my patients in the context of the following example. Allow yourself for a moment to imagine that your pain is a 600 pound rock situated in front of the door to my office. If the rock is not removed, the door will not open and I cannot see patients. In a similar manner, if you cannot remove the pain, you cannot proceed with your life. If the medical approach fails, you may incorrectly assume that it was invalid. In the greatest sense, this approach may have been correct, yet not powerful enough to move the rock. Assume that the medical approach can only exert a 200 pound pull and as a result, the rock does not move. In similar terms, both the physical and behavioral strategies applied independently are only capable of pulling 200 pounds each. Neither is strong enough to move the rock or to alleviate pain.

However, when one combines the three forces (or approaches) pulling in the same direction at precisely the same time, the rock moves and the door can be opened. Beyond just the alleviation of pain, quality of life improves for the pain sufferer. This is true synergy, the essence of *Reprogramming Pain*.

As human beings, so many factors influence the course of our lives. Unfortunately, we are not typically aware of them or their effects on us. The manner in which pain resolves or leads to chronicity can be strongly influenced by a series of occurrences, events, contacts and external influences. Many pain sufferers have basically resigned without a fight, as mere survival in this society is their ultimate goal. Even without pain, many of us tend to be overwhelmed by the challenges of day-to-day living. At some point, however, we must commit to start anew and to take control of and responsibility for our present situation. *Reprogramming Pain* was written with the belief that you have the power to positively impact your own destiny.

The most practical strategy for achieving health and happiness begins with an awareness of the mind/body relationship. The maintenance of this rather delicate balance has the potential to serve as the framework for a pain-free existence. Learning how to play a positive role in our own well-being is the most important key to living without pain.

We exist through two interrelated components called mind and body. It is impossible to separate the two functionally or structurally. They share the ultimate responsibility for the success of our continuing existence. The actions of one directly affects the other, either positively or negatively. Denying the mind/body relationship robs us of the opportunity to come to terms with and resolve ongoing pain. We must become aware of these interactions and learn how to maintain both the mind and body in a strong alliance.

Modern life in the fast lane is accompanied by persistent and intense forms of stress. If ignored or misunderstood, stress takes over and presents serious obstacles to maintaining a balanced mind/body alliance. We must learn to recognize the causes and effects of stress and become proficient in taking control of our lives.

The way we see ourselves shapes everything we do. A healthy self-image is a wonderful elixir. If you are self-confident and have a high sense of personal worth, stress is unlikely to be a major problem. If your confidence level is low and you feel that you are not in control of your life, then indeed stress, anxiety and fear become overriding feelings. The outcome is predictable and difficult to face. Ultimately, the responsibility for turning our lives around rests within ourselves.

What is pain? This question has troubled philosophers and scientists even before Aristotle. According to the 1985 National Science Foundation Research Briefing on Pain and Pain Management, "Pain has attributes of a sensation, yet its usual capacity to make us uncomfortable or to suffer distinguishes it from all other sensations." We use the term *pain* in many ways: for the feelings experienced when we are physically injured, for our emotional reactions to unkindness or loss

7

and to imply a problematic and annoying state, as in the surrendering statement, "what a pain!" The devastating element however, in chronic pain is *suffering*.

We know what pain feels like. Yet do we really understand it and, for that matter, are we aware of what it does to us? Few people realize that pain has the potential to disrupt every aspect of their existence. On a positive note, however, pain is most often self-limiting and not always an indication of poor health. More realistically, however, it is nurtured by the tension, worry or any of the other day-to-day stresses we face. No one is immune to such processes. We cannot escape the fact that the mind interacts with the body to cause and aggravate physical symptoms.

Pain takes on a new and challenging dimension when it persists. The suffering and discomfort it causes frequently destroys the quality of life for its victim. Relationships with spouse, family and friends are most vulnerable. Loss of support from our loved ones deepens the hurting. As a result, the chronic pain sufferer develops low self-worth and runs through the gauntlet of debilitating emotions: fear, guilt, helplessness, anger, frustration, loneliness and depression.

The more we hurt, the more stressed we become. Increasing stress magnifies pain and a vicious cycle ensues, which seems at times impossible to break. The elements of anxiety, depression and pain are often inseparable and their combination is like salt on an open wound. Which comes first, pain or stress? The answer is often elusive. Thus, the necessity of treating mind and body simultaneously becomes apparent.

Susan's Story

Susan, a 36-year-old secretary, has been married for 12 years and has two children. Employed full-time in a real estate firm, she enjoyed her job. Susan was active in the PTO, chairing the main fund-raising event and sharing carpooling responsibilities with other parents for dance and gymnastic lessons. Susan and her husband, Tom, both enjoyed gardening and looked forward to the time they spent together.

Fourteen months ago, Susan was involved in an automobile accident, injuring her neck. After undergoing various x-rays and scans at a local hospital, she was told that a whiplash injury (the muscles in her neck had been strained) had occurred. She was given medication for pain, fitted with a soft neck collar and was told to rest in bed for a few days and to follow up with her family doctor.

Initially, neck discomfort and occasional headaches occurred. Over time, the neck pain worsened and the frequency and severity of headaches increased. Numerous laboratory studies and scans were interpreted as normal and no physical basis was uncovered to explain her problem.

Tom and the children were very worried about Susan. They tried to be helpful and spent as much time as they could with her, attempting to lift her spirits. Despite their efforts, she became more irritable and anxious, spending more and more time in bed.

Many friends and relatives knew of doctors they were sure could help her. Susan sought the attention of several physicians, none of whom could find the cause of her pain. She was subsequently placed on a variety of medications,

9

some of which produced significant side effects, including drowsiness and depression. She consumed large quantities of coffee to keep awake. Her principal activity became watching television and for the first time since quitting 10 years ago, she began smoking. Normal eating habits changed and she started gaining weight. Susan, who had always been so meticulous about her appearance, stopped doing her hair and putting on makeup. She appeared to age considerably over the ensuing six months. The relationship with her husband deteriorated and she had little time or patience for her children. Susan lost interest in social activities and her friends stopped coming to visit. Feeling alone and becoming increasingly more depressed, Susan concluded that her very existence was meaningless and she contemplated suicide. She told her distraught husband that he and the children would be better off without her. Something had to be done to reestablish a meaningful existence.

Finally, Susan was taken to a pain clinic, more than 100 miles from her home. Initially, she was quite resistant to the evaluation, as she had basically lost confidence in the medical profession and felt a sense of being victimized. From her standpoint, she could provide little in the way of meaningful information that would help the doctors develop further insights into why her initial accident had turned into such a catastrophic event. Through a genuinely concerned and caring staff, Susan gradually began to express herself.

Eventually, it was revealed that before the accident, problems at Susan's job were causing her to feel unsettled. A branch office closed and several personnel changes occurred. A co-worker was promoted to become her manager, three associates in the office had been laid off and she was frankly worried about her own job.

Susan was frightened and she realized that a turning point in her life was likely to occur. Understandably, she was rather upset with the events that had occurred on the job. The fact that a co-worker became her manager, especially a woman who she had not gotten along with, worried her. She also realized that with this woman in charge, chances of promotion in the office were dramatically limited. To make matters worse, she was concerned with what other people would think based upon the fact that she was not promoted. Susan was inwardly disillusioned with her life, for it was not what she had expected. Despite the fact that she appeared to be a successful business woman, she was not happy with herself. Susan was extremely preoccupied with appearances and could not express her underlying fears and disappointments to her husband or to her friends.

Susan did in fact suffer a physical injury from the automobile accident 14 months ago. She did experience pain, as the muscles in her neck were truly in spasm. Unfortunately, Susan was taken off work at a crucial time and the longer she remained away from her job, the more fearful she became.

To complicate matters further, the doctors who treated her spent very little time trying to explore her psychological state. They continued to order test, after test which were repeatedly reported as negative. The frequent returning to doctors' offices to find out that the tests were normal caused Susan to slip further and further into a state of remorse and depression. The tone of communication with medical personnel seemed to indicate that the problem was most likely in her head.

Muscle relaxants and pain medications worsened matters considerably. Susan could no longer think clearly and despite her initial trust in health care providers, she became more involuted, depressed and skeptical of her doctors' judgement. One thing led to another and with a prolonged absence from work combined with a poor diet, additional caffeine, medication side effects and smoking, Susan was no longer in control of her own life. The focus of her anxiety, tension, despair and depression was placed on her neck pain and headaches, which should have improved within a rather short period of time.

If you compare Susan to the many individuals in our society who suffer in the same fashion, it becomes apparent that an initial physical injury can often turn into a nightmare and a progressive path to personal destruction. Understanding the "sacred alliance", mind/body, was the key element for improving Susan's overall state. Once her doctors focused on the inner conflicts that perpetuated her syndrome, Susan began to return to the path of health. After a three-month period of counseling and physical therapy, coupled with reassurance and a change in overall activity, Susan began to live her life anew, no longer under the cloak of pain.

David's Story

David is a tall, 38-year-old construction worker. He and his wife, Amy, have been happily married for nearly two years and plan to wait another year before starting their family.

David has always been athletic and he served as the first baseman on his company-sponsored softball team. He and his wife bowl together on a husband and wife team and love to go camping.

Six months ago, while on the job, David fell approximately five feet off a retaining wall. He immediately noted severe low back pain. David was admitted to a local hospital through the emergency room, where laboratory tests and x-rays were performed. No clear-cut abnormality was disclosed by the initial x-rays. A CT scan of his spine was ordered and again the results were negative. David was told that he had severely injured certain muscles in his back. He was placed on pain medications, muscle relaxants and complete bed rest. After four days, he was discharged from the hospital with instructions to continue taking medication as needed and to curtail all strenuous activities.

At home, David's wife cared for him but was frightened, as she had never seen him in pain before this incident. Insisting he follow the doctor's orders and stay in bed, she served all of his meals and moved the television into the bedroom. Within two weeks, he began to move about but complained that his pain was gradually worsening. He continued to ask his doctor for stronger pain medication (the dosage of the previous one had already been increased twice). The physician insisted that David be examined prior to prescribing any other pain remedy.

When they arrived at the doctor's office, Amy stayed in the waiting room. The doctor and David spoke extensively and it became apparent during the interview that David was disheartened, frustrated and depressed. He avoided his friends and family, as he was embarrassed to be seen in his present state. David was angry with his wife and stated that although he knew she meant well, she made him feel so helpless. Secretly, he believed that he was letting her down. They argued a lot and their sex life was nonexistent. He blamed his condition on the fact that, "the darn pills weren't killing the pain." Insistent that he could return to work only if the doctor would prescribe the proper drug to stop the pain, David lost sight of the true issues.

Doctor shopping for a cure failed to reveal any structural abnormality such as a fracture or dislocation. The message communicated repeatedly was that nothing was wrong physically. The last doctor frankly stated "the pain is in your head" and suggested that he seek the help of a psychiatrist. This infuriated David and he exploded in the doctor's office. The terrible pain he was experiencing was so real, yet no one would believe him. As a result, he felt totally helpless, useless, depressed and angry.

David settled into a pattern of drowning his suffering at the local bar and he often returned home drunk and angry. He would fall asleep on the couch and still be there when Amy returned home from work. When she suggested that he shower and put on clean clothes, he would become angry and tell her to stop nagging him. One night he didn't come home and Amy called some of his friends to help look for him. When they found him, David was in a rage. He told Amy he was tired of her "baby-sitting" him and that he could take care of himself.

The next evening, Amy returned home from work and David was gone. Two weeks passed without a word. Then one evening she received a call from the local police station, informing her that David had been arrested for driving while under the influence of alcohol.

Amy contacted an attorney who arranged for David's release and insisted that he seek counseling for his drinking problem before the court appearance. Through several intense sessions, David's real problem surfaced. It became apparent that David's ability to be the "bread winner" was in serious jeopardy and his self-image was severely threatened. He was also worried about the fact that many of the younger men in his company had surpassed him in their physical abilities. His fear of not measuring up as a man was compounded by the fact that x-rays, scans and an extensive medical workup indicated no fractured spine, broken bone or other REAL injury to explain his pain. He was not prepared to accept the fact that any psychological conflict could influence the pain that was so real and intense to him. Desperately, David hoped the doctors would tell him that he fractured his spine, broke a bone, tore a tendon or suffered a REAL injury. In his heart, he knew he was not faking the pain.

Before counseling, David subconsciously avoided returning to work. Prior to the accident, David began to feel his physical prowess declining and his injury was the icing on the cake. His sense of personal worth steadily declined and the longer he remained in bed, the more depressed and weakened he became. The sickening combination of pain medication and alcohol set the tone of his disposition. David was embarrassed in front of his wife and felt the only way to deal with his situation was to shut her out. Her concern and increased attention angered him and made his isolation more difficult. When it was finally suggested that David see a psychiatrist, he perceived this as the final insult to his manhood. His explosion in the doctor's office was only the initial expression of what would eventually evolve into a turbulent withdrawal.

Drinking was an escape and combined with pain medications, he lost his perspective for living. David left home, attempting to escape from his existence and was brought back to his wife after being picked up for driving under the influence of alcohol. Had it not been for the legal counsel who demanded that he seek psychological counseling, David may not have survived.

After several counseling sessions, David began the process of putting his life back together and reestablishing a more formidable bond between his mind and body. He met with a vocational counselor, entered a chronic pain management program and decided to return to school to learn a new trade. Within a period of six months, David's vistas were renewed and for the first time in several years he found peace within himself. His pain, not surprisingly, gradually disappeared.

Are We To Blame?

David is the product of a society that glorifies youth, good looks and fitness. Through the media, we learn how we are expected to appear and act. David did not begin as a drug addict. However, the promise of the "instant cure" in the form of a pill led to an ongoing addiction that contributed to his overall depression and withdrawal. This type of programming for instant relief is one of the most successful and widespread advertising themes of the century. We are taught that reaching for a pill to cure the cough, cold, aches or pain is a correct action. This belief is partially the by-product of the pharmaceutical and advertising industries that facilitate an over utilization and abuse by many susceptible individuals who are chronic pain sufferers.

David could not recapture his youth, his strength or his virility. Drinking with his friends was no longer a social habit; it became a crutch. If you review David's story, it becomes obvious that his manner of dealing with stress was "escape"; from his wife, his home, his job, his friends and from reality.

Was David's reaction unusual? The beer industry certainly thrives on the macho image David was afraid of losing. Phenomenal amounts of money are spent each year to promote such an image to the public. Linking an image to alcohol is one of the strongest and most widespread forms of conditioning in our society. Drinking a single beer for most individuals might not be considered injurious. However, the maintenance of this image, which is so widely accepted, typically does not end with just one drink. In fact, for some, drinking one beer is never enough. Conquering pain or drowning suffering is an ongoing process.

Pain may postpone or even prevent an underlying problem from surfacing. At times, pain becomes the focus of our existence and the excuse for our present condition. No doubt exists that there is a direct relationship between chronic, long-standing pain and stressful, challenging situations. The ultimate link between pain and preexisting stress is usually unknown to us and is established at the subconscious level. The end result is not accidental, as a host of external factors set the stage for such associations. Many of the ways in which we handle stress, pain or suffering are conditioned by the media, advertisers or other major industries in our society.

How many women become extremely depressed when they enter a department store in late spring to buy a bathing suit? The fashion industry links stereotyped images to their designs and their media consultants are expert at creating demand. Reality however strikes when the reflection in the dressing room mirror is quite unlike the enticing youthful look we have been programmed to admire on television. The typical woman tries on several bathing suits and walks out of the store frustrated, feeling incompetent, overweight and unhappy with herself. The perfect body image does not provide a realistic model for the average woman; it promotes a sense of failure and diminished self-worth.

Frequently, we feel inadequate because the product does not fit. We do not live up to the image that we admire on television and as a result, learn to drown our programmed sense of reality with cigarettes or alcohol. In a similar manner, we are not taught to face pain in an objective fashion or to develop a better understanding of the mind/body alliance. Reaching for a pill to produce the instant cure is no more than a programmed response. We are not encouraged to be introspective, to talk about our problems or to deal with issues. We are expected to maintain a role or an image, patterned by those who do not have our best interests at heart.

The media is not the only culprit. The traditional medical model conditions us to believe that if a bone is not broken, a significant problem does not exist. We are often disappointed to receive the news of a normal x-ray or negative scan which serves as an indication that there is no physical problem. The physician's manner of explanation often inadvertently suggests that the problem is inconsequential and the patient's need to understand pain is often ignored. Some practitioners do not take the time to discuss these issues with their patients. They use phrases such as "there is nothing wrong" or "maybe its your nerves," instead of taking the time to openly and supportively discuss the sacred alliance: mind and body. This lack of empathy is one of the most substantial forms of negative societal conditioning, which can potentially induce or worsen a pattern of psychobiological distress. Such deficiencies in physician-patient communications may result in irreparable consequences.

The best way to effectively deal with these issues is to better understand the true nature of pain in terms of a mind/body alliance. We must establish a realistic frame of reference in order to recognize the programming messages we are bombarded with throughout our lives. The next chapter will unravel the basis for pain and the mystery of this sacred alliance.

Chapter 2

The Origins of Pain

The Brain-Body Circuit

Somewhere along the evolutionary process, pain's basic protective circuitry became interwoven with other neural circuits to produce a system encroaching upon almost every aspect of human function and behavior.

Even primitive organisms protect themselves. It is not surprising that human evolution proceeded with the corresponding development of basic pain systems necessary for life-sustaining and protective activities. As man's development progressed through the ages, the anatomical, biochemical and functional basis for pain became predictably more complex and began to serve him on different levels. Somewhere along the evolutionary process, pain's basic protective circuitry became interwoven with other neural circuits to produce a system intertwined with almost every aspect of human function and behavior. Throughout the ages, man has tried to comprehend this all-encompassing system. Despite notable advances in medical science and technology, our understanding of the way we process pain is most certainly incomplete.

The Brain As A Computer

Human pain processes can be superficially described as analogous to the operations of a modern day computer. Let's take a moment to explore how a computer system works. Data flows into the system through a keyboard which, for our purposes, represents a series of specific sensory receptors. Just as each key signifies a different letter or number, different neural sensors are similarly specialized. Pressing one key on a keyboard sends a coded message to the computer which it interprets as a specific character. In a similar manner, stimulating a specific body receptor sends a code that the brain may read as a painful stimulus.

The nervous system consists of two respective components: the peripheral and the central nervous system. Basically, sensors and nerves leading to and emerging from the spinal cord constitute the peripheral nervous system. The brain and spinal cord are referred to as the central nervous system. This analogy extends to our computer model as well. Both the keyboard and computer screen are seen as the peripheral system and the computer itself should be considered as equivalent to the central nervous system.

Pain receptors are specialized neural elements, sometimes just bare nerve endings in the skin, along specific key anatomical points. Often, pain signals are transmitted along the paths of nerves that primarily serve other bodily functions. These fibers typically terminate in the spinal cord or brain stem. Compare these connections to the keyboard cable that plugs into the computer. Every wire has its place and similarly, each nerve fiber is destined to end in a specific location within the central nervous system.

Nerves send messages by electrical and chemical means. Impulses may pass along a nerve surface or skip segments, based on the organization of the insulation or myelin coating. The speed of conducted impulses can often serve to identify the type of stimulus present. Nerve fiber types have been classified by size, coating and speed of conduction. This organization provides the basis for signal coding that may be altered in diseased states or as the result of certain types of injury.

Like computer keys, sensory nerve endings maintain different functions and have the potential to send a variety of messages. Under normal circumstances, it is a straightforward task for the organism to discriminate touch, vibration, pain or position, technically referred to as proprioception. The ability to differentiate these sensations is partially the result of receptor type and location. It is important to realize that the integrity of the nervous system depends to a large extent on the overall health of the organism.

The density of nerve endings or sensors in a given location varies with function. Sensitive regions of the body are characterized by an increased number of fibers. You would expect increased numbers of fibers in areas such as the finger tips, as the ability to perform fine motor tasks such as repairing a watch or painting a picture depends on the ability to sense fine changes. Regions such as the forearms or the chest wall are less sensitive and contain lower fiber densities.

Let's return to our example of the computer. Suppose for a moment that the spinal cord is comparable to a printed circuit board. Wires leading from the computer keyboard attach via the plug to the computer's printed circuit board and are subsequently redirected to specific components. By similar means, the peripheral sensory nerves for pain enter the spinal cord at various levels and are precisely channeled to other spinal levels or to specific areas of the brain through its stalk, the brain stem.

Computer wires are soldered to the circuit board and to each other for precise connections. Unlike these wires, nerves lie in close proximity to other nerves in a specific pathway or tract, but they never touch each other or establish physical contact. Information is transferred through the microscopic space between the nerves called the "synapse," where the chemistry of the nervous system takes over and precisely controls the transmission of impulses from one region to another. The synapse is truly one of the most important centers for control of the pain circuit.

The chemicals that flow across the synapse are termed "neurotransmitters" and medical scientists specifically design medications to affect this portion of the circuit. It is interesting to note that certain medicines and hormones affect specialized synapses, which vary according to location and neurotransmitter type. Several different types of synapses have been discovered and our knowledge of neurotransmitters is expanding at a phenomenal rate. Take a moment to imagine the complexity of a pain circuit with thousands of synapses simultaneously controlling an incredible flow of information and operating under the precise control of several potent chemical messengers.

Getting back to our computer model, it's important to remember that even when the keystroke is recognized by a computer, nothing much has been accomplished. Your budget has not been balanced, your day has not been scheduled and your data has not been analyzed. In the same manner, sending pain signals to the central nervous system represents only the beginning of our pain circuit. An accumulation of a series of specific key strokes is of course necessary before the computer can perform a meaningful task. The series of steps necessary to organize and decipher data is termed *processing*. This important function is accomplished under the control of a series of instructions designed for a specific purpose and termed the *program*. Without this instructional set, the computer would be left with a series of meaningless letters and numbers. Such necessary steps are carried out by the computer's central processing unit or CPU.

The central nervous system's CPU is the brain. It is here that pain signals are processed, interpreted and attached to feelings and behavior. Complex circuitry is involved and biochemical reactions proceed in a microscopic system containing large numbers of neurons. The brain's detail, circuitry and precision, coupled with its ability to perform literally millions of simultaneous interactions is amazing. The potential for programming a system with such inherent complexity is beyond the realm of comprehension. The world's most advanced computers have stunned us with their capabilities, yet they do not even come close to approaching the potential of a human brain. It's not surprising that in such a complex and advanced neurological system, even the slightest anatomical or chemical change can lead to considerable variations in overall behavior.

If we trace pain impulses through the central nervous system, the journey would traverse many important structures and relay stations between the original receptors and the brain. Projections of nerve fiber extend through central collections of nerves cells such as the thalamus (located in the forebrain) and settle along the edges of the brain in specially demarcated functional zones, called Brodmann's areas. More than 50 such zones are known to exist. These areas, which have been mapped and studied over the years, also send fibers to other specific integrative regions and functional zones. The volley of information between these areas is constant.

The human brain, not unlike the central processing unit of a computer, can be divided into specialized regions that are functionally related. It appears that the brain's functional development paralleled a logical evolutionary process, just as the computer's CPU has been progressively refined to dedicate specific areas to functions such as video processing, sound control and recognition of what enters and exits the system.

The somatosensory cortex, a specialized ribbon of nerve cells on the edge of the brain is an important structure for the projection of sensory fibers. The most basic information in the path of a pain impulse settles in this location, detecting and partially identifying the origin of the signal.

Pain impulses reaching this area are projected to mapped areas within the brain corresponding to the body's anatomy. Body parts that are highly sensitive have a larger representation on the somatosensory cortex. The first individuals to discover this natural wiring diagram were the Greeks who believed that a miniature man (homunculus) was located inside of a sperm. They projected the image of an upside down homunculus with disproportionately large lips and hands on the outer surface of the brain, in order to explain the regional mapping of neural signals. Even today, this basic understanding of surface maps in the brain is accepted. Unfortunately, many of the components of pain have not been deciphered.

Simply determining the type of impulse received and recognizing its origin provides little benefit for an organism. Even though a computer may identify a keystroke as a letter, it cannot perform any particularly meaningful function with just that data. In a similar manner, peripheral pain information is of no practical use without brain processing through specific neural programs.

A Theoretical Creature

Let's explore the nervous system of a simple fictional animal that we will take the liberty to design and call a "LOUIE." The extent of this animal's evolution is primitive and its principle life-sustaining functions are limited. Louie has the ability to breathe, eat and reproduce--no more and no less. Assume that breathing is basically automatic and for the purposes of our discussion, let's not focus on reproduction.

He is unemotional, cannot be offended and does not have the capacity to hold a grudge. Louie eats bugs, which are not always found in his immediate vicinity. Walking on all fours, he spends a great deal of time finding food for survival. Louie has a relatively uncomplicated, primitive pain system, unassociated with highly developed emotions. Let's follow our furry friend through the forest to develop a better understanding of basic pain mechanisms.

After a relaxing day basking in the sun, Louie decides to find food. Strolling through the forest, he finds a fly here or there but nothing substantial enough to serve as a hearty meal. He enters a thicket (his vision is not well developed) and stubs his toe. Up to this point, life has been simple but, alas, the pain cycle now begins.

A receptor, actually just a bare nerve ending in Louie's foot, is sensitive to pain and when stimulated, sends a message to the spinal column. Through a primitive reflex response actually controlled in the spinal cord, certain muscles in the injured leg are activated while others simultaneously relax, as the limb is automatically withdrawn. Other circuits are swiftly called into action and muscles of the opposite leg immediately contract in order to stabilize our poor friend to prevent a fall. This happens in a split second. Our little creature is saved for the moment.

If these actions represented the highest level of neural development, Louie would accomplish no more than withdrawing the toe and stabilizing his body. Even our primitive friend needs to learn something from his painful ordeal. It's important to understand that, to this point, we have focused our attention only upon the most rudimentary mechanisms of pain behavior.

After his initial reflex response, nerve impulses travel to the brain, passing through some interesting regions (which we'll get back to later) and settling in Louie's basic pain cortex. This brain region detects the stimulus and localizes it to the left toe. So far, the organism has only recognized and responded to pain. If no further cerebral processing occurs, Louie would be in trouble. Fortunately, even for our simple-minded creature, that's not the case.

Those interesting brain areas alluded to previously are extremely important for survival. Pain signals are transmitted to "association areas" in the brain, where they are processed into useful information. Louie already knows he is in pain. However, the association areas are necessary to recognize what these signals mean. Eventually, a limited memory bank (sorry Louie!) attaches dangerous connotations to the stubbing of his toe. In effect, Louie's central nervous system allows him to realize that this is bad news.

Even a simple subject like Louie needs to learn about pain in order to survive. There are only so many times he can be injured without a major catastrophe. Louie must learn to not enter the thicket and his memory bank must be loaded with data about the forest floor and the environment in general. However, these memories alone, established via specific neural circuits, are not enough to produce defensive pain behavior sufficient to help Louie survive. More complex functions must be called into action to begin the process of recognizing potential sources of pain and avoiding them. Even our simpleton must evolve further. Let's spend a few moments exploring this process on human terms.

The Anatomical and Chemical Basis
For Pain Behavior

Neural circuits establish connections with specific association, sensory and memory areas for the purpose of integrat-
ing feelings, insights, speculations and personal direction.
In addition to pain sensors, we utilize our senses of vision,
hearing, smell, taste and touch to develop more complex
pain behaviors. We are programmed through visual stimuli
to slam the foot on the brake to avoid a collision. In a
similar manner, a state of protective arousal automatically
occurs, causing us to flee from the smell of a burning building. These actions help to ensure the survival of a person.

Unfortunately, sensory associations are not always helpful
and sometimes they cause pain. Seeing the image in your
mind of someone who may have hurt you in the past can
reactivate severe back pain and spasm. Although a specific
perfume may evoke a state of heightened sexual arousal,
that same fragrance, when associated with a painful divorce
can induce abdominal pain. These types of associations are
far-reaching, deeply programmed and not always obvious.
Understanding the phenomenal complexities of supposedly
protective neural circuits is vastly beyond our present scope
of knowledge. Yet the issues surrounding them are very important when we attempt to understand the mind/body connection.

To complicate matters further, let's get back to those
microscopic spaces between the nerves called synapses. It
is here that the biochemistry of pain resides. The experiencing of emotions, sensations and physical actions all re-

lease different chemicals into our bodies. The brain and the central nervous system have an amazing capacity to recognize and react to a huge variety of different chemical combinations. The modulating substances of pain are called neurotransmitters and the locations of these chemicals are often found, not surprisingly, in rather specific areas of the nervous system and body. For example, serotonin, one of the prime neurotransmitters associated with pain, is highly localizable to the Dorsal Raphe Nucleus, an area of the brain thought by some to be the seat of migraine headaches. Interestingly enough, one of the highest concentrations of serotonin exists in the gut. Does it surprise you that some of migraine's most commonly related symptoms are nausea and vomiting? Have you ever thought about that sinking feeling in your stomach before a dental visit? These symptoms and feelings are predictable and are neurochemically mediated.

Depression, sleep disruption and muscle aches are often accompanying complaints for migraine sufferers. Similar types of medicine are utilized to treat all of these problems and serotonin is thought to be a potential common culprit. One of the most poorly understood, yet ridiculed disorders in our society is PMS or premenstrual syndrome. Many medical professionals and laymen alike believe that the complaints of PMS are no more than psychological fabrications. Just consider for a moment that a woman describing her symptoms mentions feelings of depression, headaches, muscle cramps, gastric distress and difficulty sleeping. It certainly sounds like a problem associated with serotonin metabolism. Medical scientists have learned that changes in female hormonal levels directly affect the binding of se-rotonin to the nerve ending. The neurotransmitter is present and it crosses the synapse, but it doesn't get bound to the necessary site. As a result, the essential nerve impulse is not properly conducted--hence the development of PMS!

Other synaptic considerations are necessary to help provide a better understanding of pain. Some synapses can be *excitatory* and others are *inhibitory*. Excitatory synapses, when stimulated, facilitate the transmission of a message to the next nerve in the circuit. Inhibitory ones impede or block the flow of information. Of importance is the fact that only a certain amount of data can traverse a synapse in a given period of time. In the mid-1960s, neuro-scientists began to entertain the theory of a spinal cord sys-tem that could, under certain conditions, either allow a pain signal to proceed along its course or stop it in its tracks. This model was coined the "Gate Theory" by Melzak and Wall. In its simplest form, the theory presumes that certain forms of stimuli to the skin can overload the system with messages to a specific spinal cord locus where, under cer-tain conditions, the transmission of an actual pain signal can be blocked. Suppose for a moment that you are experi-encing pain from a strained muscle in the low back. If a set of electrodes is placed over the painful area and low inten-sity electrical pulses are delivered to the skin through a por-table battery-operated device, the perception of the original back pain could be blocked by overloading the original pain circuit. This device is the modern day TENS, or transcuta-neous nerve stimulation unit, frequently utilized as a popu-lar form of therapy for pain control. Acupuncture is thought

32

by some to represent another example of a pain control system operating via the Gate Theory.

A Closer Look at the Mind-Body Continuum

The body's own chemically mediated pain control mechanisms have become a major source of interest over the last 20 or so years, as people began to focus on natural healing methods for pain. Pain controlling substances, termed *endorphins*, are known to play an important role in the modulation and control of pain. The study of endorphins and their binding sites has progressed to the present day understanding of the existence of several distinct peptides or proteins found in specific anatomical regions of the spinal cord, brain and body. Some of these substances, which are referred to as neuropeptides, serve as the body's own morphine-like substances.

Many studies have described changes in the levels of endorphins induced by activities such as acupuncture, TENS, biofeedback, exercise, meditation, hypnosis and stress. It is believed that the "runner's high" is based upon the body's production of these endorphins. Despite a universal interest in these substances, their structure and biochemistry has not yet been fully disclosed. In addition, peptides such as Substance P are becoming the center of focus in a large number of studies concerning chemical mediation of pain pathways. The release of these substances is being explored from the perspective of developing agents to enhance or block conduction in these circuits.

33

In essence, it has been postulated that emotional responses exist based upon the release of certain peptides and the coupling of these agents with specific receptors found almost everywhere in the body. Referring to these substances in *Healing and The Mind*, Dr. Candace Pert, a world-renowned psychoneuroimmunologist, stated, "They seem to be extremely important because they appear to mediate intercellular communication throughout the brain and body." She proceeded to state, "We have come to theorize that these neuropeptides and their receptors are the biological correlates of emotion." Dr. Pert's remarkable findings have narrowed the search for the mind/body alliance to the cellular level. Future investigations will better define the roles of neural peptides in the pain circuit.

The Autonomic Nervous System

Pain's neural connections are vast and probably relate to more aspects of human function than ever imagined. Pain affects both voluntary and involuntary body systems. Perhaps its most interesting impact is on the autonomic or supposedly automatic nervous system (ANS). The ANS regulates specific activities of the heart, blood vessels, respiratory system, glands, digestive tract, bladder and sexual organs. Many of these functions thought to be entirely automatic in the past, are now known to be controllable at will.

As previously implied, some of the brain's circuitry evolved with crossovers to other systems. The ramifications of these evolved circuits are not always positive. The "fight or flight" response, characterized by autonomic activation, yields dilated pupils, increased sweating, rapid heart rate, elevated blood pressure, changes in blood flow and a heightened state of arousal. This highly studied response basically serves as a protective and preparatory reaction to a threatening situation. This response is extremely important in humans, as chronic pain and prolonged stress induces autonomic changes that can be responsible for the deterioration of the overall health of an individual. Pain circuitry is so closely associated with autonomic pathways that such responses can sometimes become the hallmark of a painful process. Despite the fact that these automatic responses are meant to protect organisms from danger, they may induce high blood pressure, respiratory problems, gastrointestinal distress and even heart attacks. At times, the autonomic nervous system becomes an unpredictable villain in the development of some of the most challenging pain syndromes. Sometimes autonomic involvement produces diminished regional blood flow to a limb, associated with a severe, burning sensation, unpredictable skin temperature changes, swelling and excruciating pain on movement. This pattern of symptoms is termed Reflex Sympathetic Dystrophy or RSD. When one considers this example and the vast integration of pain circuitry with other brain systems, it's not surprising to note that a person experiencing a chronic pain syndrome often suffers on many levels.

A relatively new field, Psychoneuroimmunology, is evolving. "Psycho" refers to the mind, "neuro" to the nervous system and "immunology" to the study of the body's defense mechanisms against infection. A number of studies have shown that stress affects the body's immune potential to fight infections. It has been demonstrated that college students suffer more respiratory infections when under the stress of final exams. It is not unusual to find a patient in chronic pain, fighting off infection after infection, despite multiple antibiotic regimens.

The application of such knowledge can also produce positive and healthful results. Dr. Lee Berk, of Loma Linda University, one of the foremost researchers of our time in the field of Psychoneuroimmunology, has clearly demonstrated that laughter can reproducibly improve immune function. His hallmark work represents only the beginning of what appears to be one of the most promising areas of science. The understanding of the mind's role in immune function has the potential to improve dramatically the quality of life on this planet.

One could write an entire text on almost every component of this chapter. The specialization of the nervous system is so complex that distinct disciplines within the neurosciences have emerged in order to focus on very specific elements. Yet despite such an extensive fund of knowledge, our understanding of the subject is truly in its infancy. This chapter only briefly touched on some of the important components necessary for the understanding of pain syndromes. It serves as a limited introduction for a series of insights to be covered in later chapters.

Chapter 3

The Mind's Role

The Invisible Navigator

*Our concept of pain is so deeply pro-
grammed that it becomes impossible
to separate the hurt from a lifetime
of accumulated associations.*

A ship destined to sail must be designed to
enable its purpose. Its sails, fittings and lines
are basic and necessary components. Yet in
the final analysis, the overall success of the
voyage depends on the captain's ability to
navigate the vessel safely through the oceans.

The prior chapter's explanation of pain receptors, circuitry and chemistry oversimplifies one of the most complex functions of the human body. Pain mechanisms are
modulated by complex neural interactions that have the potential to produce a state of being that can overwhelm an
individual. The voyage of living with pain is truly under the
control of the "invisible navigator," the mind.

Human development evolves through a wide variety of experiences and learning processes. From birth, we are programmed to respond in certain ways and to interact with our environment in set patterns. Of course, genetics plays an important role in our responsiveness to external influences. Programming our genetic base has been demonstrated to produce predictable and characteristic responses.

An individual's manner of suffering is unique to that person. It is based on a lifetime of programming. Understanding one's expression of chronic pain is complex, as pain behavior is no less complicated than an individual's existence. It cannot be deciphered easily.

How do you describe a person? Is it by appearance, height, weight, age, skin color, ethnic origin or education? Even after studying these details, you know little about the individual. It's obvious that the most important aspects of their being have not surfaced. Similarly, blood pressure, pulse, reflexes and degree of muscle spasm reveal little about a person suffering from an overwhelming and chronic pain syndrome. The key to helping a person in chronic pain may lie in understanding the complexity of his or her existence. We can begin by exploring the mind's influence on the body and the body's influence on the mind.

To complicate matters further, it is not only the patient's experiential background that must be taken into account, the programming of the health care provider is a major factor in treatment as well. The health care provider's personal background and professional conditioning often contributes to a sea of confusion. The interaction between patient and doctor may be one of the most critical factors to be addressed in reestablishing a pain-free existence.

As children, we learn complex lessons in simple ways. Touching a hot burner produces a reflex reaction, an avoidance response that will last a lifetime. Such an imprint on the memory center not only exists for a specific event, but is often reverberated on demand and triggered by other experiences. Painful and pleasurable associations are developed very early on. Even with minimal experience, children learn rather early how to control their environments. A kiss on the forehead or a mother's hug after a bruise to the knee establishes a powerful and far reaching imprint that lasts indefinitely.

External programming also results in memory imprints. That great-looking actor on television who "bangs back the pain" produces a remarkable influence on the viewers, one that serves as the financial backbone of a multimillion dollar industry. Most individuals do not realize the incredible programming power of a kiss on the forehead or a well-planned television commercial. The message to avoid pain at any cost is repeated over and over on television, on billboards, in magazines and newspapers and becomes a programmed subconscious reaction, leading us to reach for the pill that will immediately eliminate our pain. We progress from the kiss that makes it all better to the latest drug for instant relief. It's commonplace for most advertisers to present a caring parent or spouse giving the latest remedy to an ailing loved-one. Do not be lured into believing that this association is coincidental.

It has been stated that medical schools often emphasize the role of becoming an objective scientist at the expense of practicing the art of medicine. Even with such training, a caregiver can usually spot an emotional individual. However, lack of insight may result in communications with a patient that are interpreted as being delivered with demeaning and disconcerting overtones. Given the respect most of us have for our physicians, it should come as no surprise that the manner in which we are treated can often influence our progress.

Two Of A Kind

Jonathan is a 42-year-old engineer who went to his doctor for the treatment of recurring headaches. He described his pain as a tightening and aching sensation and mentioned no other symptoms. His examination revealed no abnormal findings and his doctor believed that the problem was most likely related to "musculoskeletal" or "tension," headaches.

Maria is a 26-year-old housewife who sought the attention of the same physician. She complained of an intense, searing, vice-like, squeezing headache, associated with nausea, profound light-headedness and heaviness of her head. She also described related symptoms including anxiety, fatigue, frustration and worry. Her examination was noted to be entirely normal. Maria's diagnosis was "neurosis with emotionally based headaches."

The descriptions of Jonathan's and Maria's headaches were quite different. The first appeared to be objective, unassociated with any clear-cut emotional overlay. The second revealed an intense emotional component. Since Jonathan's description of pain was unemotional, the doctor accepted it at face value and prescribed a straightforward treatment regimen incorporating anti-inflammatory medications and a muscle relaxant. Maria expressed distress and anxiety and the physician accepted her actions as an expression of a psychosomatic disorder. Her headaches were treated with sedatives or calming agents.

Although the physician's impressions were different, by diagnostic criteria, the headaches were essentially the same. The difference in diagnosis resulted from the patients' descriptions of their symptoms. Of importance, however, is the fact that the physician diagnosed and treated the individuals differently. Jonathan was not considered hysterical or "psychosomatic" until after three or four attempts with pharmacological therapy, his headaches persisted and other potential contributing factors surfaced.

If we theoretically inflicted a specific painful stimulus on a group of people, a host of different responses would be elicited. Emotional factors from the present or past would play an important role in how pain was perceived and described. If we are relaxed or composed, a painful stimulus could be viewed as nonthreatening and the description might be somewhat objective. However, if we are frightened or worried, that same stimulus could certainly produce a profoundly different response, possibly suggestive of substantial psychological overlay.

We recently surveyed a number of our colleagues and asked for words associated with pain. The responses ranged from *abuse* to *worry*. As we suspected, many emotions appeared to be associated with the word *pain*. These included anxiety, avoidance, crankiness, depression, disgust, distress, empathy, fatigue, frustration, heartache, loneliness, nagging, sorrow and worry. It became apparent after reviewing the responses, that words associated with pain did not so much describe the sensation, but rather indicated feelings, events or activities related to painful experiences.

The word *pain* takes on a variety of meanings under different circumstances and descriptions of it often act as a barometer of our emotional state. Our pain vocabulary can be extremely revealing and it serves as a reflection of our inner workings. Spend a few moments to list 10 words you associate with pain. We will call this list your Reprogramming Pain Inventory (RPI). Later today, review your list (pretend it's about someone else) and try to visualize an individual whom these words might describe. Show your RPI to a friend or loved-one and ask him or her to do the same. The results could be fascinating and surprising! Through this simple exercise, you can begin to develop phenomenal insights and learn a great deal about yourself and others. The words you choose and the images they summon probably say more about your life than about the sensation of pain.

Individuals suffering from chronic pain frequently lose sight of the actual feeling itself. Awakening with a sick, unrested feeling associated with hopelessness and depression may actually be what many pain sufferers refer to as pain. Descriptions of such physical conditions are sometimes vague and may reflect an overall state of being that becomes the worst pain of all; existence without hope. Our concept of pain is so deeply programmed that separating the hurt from a lifetime of accumulated associations and feelings is impossible.

The mind is frequently programmed through the spoken word. It is therefore important to understand the relationship between a word and its meaning. The notion of attempting to characterize pain by the patient's description is often difficult. The manner of expression, or body language, rather than pain itself, can in many ways uncover clues about the person. Diagnosing the basis for a painful condition, considering purely descriptive phrases rather than attempting to take the time to understand the sufferer, often results in predictable failure.

Misconceptions concerning the basis for pain may also foster detrimental sentiments. If an individual believes that pain is associated with a nerve root being squashed, pinched or compressed, the visual image developed in the subconscious sometimes produces a defensive and fearful emotional posture. Often, failure to understand the physical nature of an injury produces misinterpretations with detrimental emotional consequences. Furthermore, physicians may increase overall anxiety by using terms that are not readily understandable. The caretaker's words are powerful and may perpetuate pain and suffering. Terms such as *strained, stretched, torn* or *injured* are perceived in different ways. An ongoing pain syndrome can be programmed through the use of intimidating terminology and a diagnosis may take on a meaning that was never intended by the physician.

Jennifer's Story

Jennifer is a 29-year-old account executive for a major publishing firm. While vacationing on a holiday weekend, she was thrown from a horse and suffered a few minor scrapes and bruises. After getting back on the saddle, she began to notice tightness in her neck. By the following morning, severe pain and spasm developed, prompting a visit to an emergency room. After waiting three hours, she underwent a series of x-rays and a short medical exam. No fracture was noted and the nurse relayed the doctor's orders for a muscle relaxant and pain killer. Jennifer was anxious about the pain and questioned the nurse, who suggested she had a *pinched* nerve that would improve in a few days. She was asked to follow-up with her family physician.

After taking medication faithfully for three days, Jennifer became concerned that the pain had not subsided. Her family doctor agreed with the diagnosis of a *pinched* nerve and tried to reassure her that the problem would take care of itself. Jennifer's pain progressively worsened, and she began to take more medication in an effort to continue working. Weakness and fatigue set in, and her mood became more somber. One morning, she awoke in a cold sweat, breathing rapidly and experiencing numbness in her hands and lips. Based upon these new symptoms, a scan was ordered by an emergency room physician to rule out a spinal cord compression. She returned home, fearful, depressed and awaiting a call to return for surgery. The next day, her family doctor called and stated that she had a *bulging* disc in her neck and a consultation with a neurosurgeon was scheduled.

Life for Jennifer was a nightmare while she anticipated the dreaded visit. By the day of the appointment, she was extremely traumatized and the neurosurgeon was confronted by an hysterical woman. He agreed that the disc was *bulging* but refused to operate, curtly stating that surgery was not indicated. His suggestion to visit a psychiatrist was met with anger, frustration and despair. For the next three months, Jennifer did not return to work and eventually she lost her job, became more recluse and lost 25 pounds. A subsequent disability examination performed by an orthopedic surgeon failed to reveal a physical basis for her complaints. Having given up, she moved back to her parents' home.

A recommendation from her mother's best friend prompted an appointment with an osteopathic anesthesiologist pain-management specialist, who worked at a local center. After a thorough history and physical examination, the doctor proceeded to review her spinal x-rays and CT scan. He presented a diagnosis of Fibromyalgia, carefully explaining that her muscles were in spasm and that the x-rays were normal.

Jennifer immediately challenged the diagnosis and told him that he had missed a *bulging* disc and a *pinched* nerve. The anesthesiologist calmly discussed his findings, explaining that *bulging* discs were commonly found in many individuals without pain syndromes. He proceeded to demonstrate similar findings on other scans and provided her with two comprehensive pamphlets on the subject. Although reluctant to part with her prior diagnosis, Jennifer agreed to try a different approach.

After a short series of local muscle injections, coupled with a collaborative pain management program that included appropriate medications, massage, physical therapy, biofeedback and counseling, Jennifer's veil of pain began to lift. Within three months, her depression, solitude and remorse gradually faded, and she regained the quality of life she had previously enjoyed.

Jennifer's story is not uncommon. Many people develop heightened suffering out of misunderstanding or fear. Her problem actually began in the emergency room when the doctor was too busy to explain his findings and the x-ray report. When the nurse relayed the message that the diagnosis was a *"pinched* nerve," Jennifer created a mental image of a sensitive nerve squeezed in a vice of bone against bone. Her family doctor did not spend sufficient time explaining the problem or the prognosis, nor did he explain a realistic course of events. Her lack of progress was interpreted as a sign of a more serious underlying problem. His terminology only reinforced her misunderstanding. When Jennifer awoke in a cold sweat with rapid breathing and numb hands, she was most likely suffering from an anxiety attack coupled with hyperventilation. However, in her confusion and fear, she associated all of her symptoms with her accident. In her mind, the initial injury was becoming more serious.

When it was suggested that Jennifer consult a neurosurgeon, she was further convinced that her fears were justifiable and that she was seriously injured. Rather than explaining that a *bulging* disc is often a common finding with no associated clinical consequence, the neurosurgeon appeared to brush her off as a neurotic. If he had taken the time to explain that a nerve was not crushed, pinched or damaged, she may not have developed the subsequent problems. Instead, she left the surgeon's office believing that she was incurable and deserved a visit to the local shrink.

Jennifer was programmed deleteriously from the start. Eventually she met a supportive and open-minded physician, who gave her a realistic explanation and a new chance.

We must always take into account that misinformation or lack of understanding can lead to tragic consequences. Information delivered in an uncaring manner is even more likely to be misunderstood or distorted by a frightened patient. This problem extends beyond the attitudes of health care providers and enters into every aspect of our lives.

The complaint of pain often influences those around us and preconceived notions often generate a host of new issues and problems. Let's explore the following scenario. When you are sick in bed with a horrible headache and cannot get to work, it is not considered prudent to call the office and say, "I have a headache." This is not a good move. We are programmed to accept symptoms such as fever, chills, vomiting and diarrhea as legitimate medical excuses for staying home. After all, no boss wants you to present to work in that condition. *Headache*, however, carries a different connotation. Calling in with a headache is unlikely to be a well-tolerated action. Non headache sufferers simply do not understand the debilitating effects of this type of pain. It is not surprising that the estimated number of days lost from work secondary to headaches represents a gross underestimate. Just imagine the true financial impact on our industrialized society from this disorder alone.

The seeds for our perceptions and reactions to pain are planted in our minds very early in our lives. As we grow and interact with society, our pain interpretation mechanisms evolve. Primary pain responses are often modified by the people with whom we identify, our education and our experiences. It is safe to say that no two people perceive pain in precisely the same manner. Unfortunately, the memory of past painful experiences or associated feelings may have more adverse effects on a medical condition than present circumstances. Uncovering such a phenomenon can be extremely difficult.

Dan's Story

Dan is a 19-year-old sophomore at an Ivy League university on the East coast. He always enjoyed good health and played soccer and lacrosse. An excellent student, Dan distinguished himself as captain of the debating team in his second collegiate year.

One day, while jogging with a friend, Dan tripped and struck his head on a cement planter. After briefly losing consciousness, Dan awoke dazed and unclear about what had happened to him. A friend called an ambulance and Dan was taken to a local hospital emergency room, where he underwent a work-up, which included a scan of the brain and an EEG (brain wave test). Dan was told by the doctor that he suffered a minor concussion and needed to stay overnight for observation. He awoke the next morning with nausea and vomiting. The physician and the nursing staff reassured him that his present symptoms were consistent with this diagnosis. Nausea and vomiting ensued for another two days and he was not discharged until the end of the week.

When he returned to the dorm, Dan's friends noticed a change. He appeared quiet, complained of headaches and was light-headed. No longer able to read for hours on end, his grades precipitously dropped, and he became disinterested in extracurricular activities. By the end of the semes-

ter, despite the use of many pain medications, Dan continued to manifest headaches and was forced to take a leave
from school.

Upon his arrival home, Dan's distraught parents took
him to see their family physician. After a complete examination, which was described as being normal, the doctor
ordered another series of x-rays and scans, all of which were
negative. Unable to find the cause of Dan's pain, the doctor referred him to a local neurologist.

The neurologist examined and talked briefly with Dan,
telling him that he was suffering from posttraumatic headaches. He prescribed various medications, none of which
helped. Six months later, Dan spoke with another physician
who suggested a psychologist who used biofeedback therapy.
After a few sessions, Dan began to develop a knack for
self-relaxation and his headaches improved to a moderate
degree. The psychologist asked Dan to consider any inner
conflicts or possible subconscious blocks that could have
been preventing his return to health. None immediately surfaced.
Dan eventually agreed to undergo a series of hypnosis sessions, which ultimately revealed that his grandfather, with
whom he had been very close, fell off a riding lawn mower
one Sunday afternoon when Dan was six. Under hypnosis,
he recalled running over to his grandfather and frantically
trying to wake him. The image of a pool of blood pouring
from the unconscious man's nose had apparently been bur-
ied deeply in his subconscious. He watched as his closest
friend, his grandfather, died of a brain hemorrhage.

Dan had always been haunted by the pain of this event
without knowing it. His fall reactivated feelings that were

progressively destroying his life. Unable to initially justify his light-headedness and headaches, Dan, through counseling sessions, became aware of the devastating link between his present and past suffering. His symptoms gradually disappeared, and he progressively became able to restore balance in his life and return to school. Dan's "invisible navigator" led him on a painful voyage.

Pain on Pain

Pain influences our perception. Experiencing an abscessed tooth, fracture or an episode of facial neuralgia can lead to a permanent imprint in the brain's memory center. Patients with chronic pain syndromes most often appear depressed and one can erroneously assume that their pain is purely psychological. The familiarity of the condescending statement, "it's all in your head," indicates the lack of seriousness given to the psychological effects of pain. Some people actually believe that nothing cures depression like a good dose of pain.

Imagine awakening with a severe headache six months ago. By noon, the discomfort crescendoes to an insurmountable level and nausea and vomiting develops. By evening, the pain gradually resolves. Suppose that after six months another headache develops. It's conceivable that you would simply take a few over-the-counter pain pills and proceed to work as usual, hoping that the pain would disappear.

Contrast this with an individual who experienced the same type of headache you did six months ago and who awakes with similar headaches three days out of each week on a regular basis. It is inconceivable to expect that individual to function normally. After repeated and predictable episodes, that person would awaken, note the onset of a headache and undergo a classic series of mental reactions; anger, despair, frustration and depression. Adrenaline would flow, muscles would tighten, blood pressure would rise and these physical responses would serve to worsen or perpetuate the headache. Is this series of events reflective of a psychiatric illness?

The answer is no. The response is a normal one, programmed by experience. If a rat is placed in a maze and receives a shock each time it enters a specific corridor, it quickly learns to anticipate the punishment and will take another route. In the same fashion, we learn to expect a horrible headache if certain symptoms are present on a repetitive basis. Just the memory of a supposedly unavoidable experience programs a specific and often detrimental central nervous system response. It is important to understand that ongoing pain perpetuates itself.

We must realize that pain behavior is strongly influenced by our families, friends and loved-ones. The mind is extremely receptive to such external influences that are sometimes overwhelming. The following case history demonstrates the importance of considering the influence of family members on the development of pain behavior.

Jason's Story

Jason is a bright yet quiet 10-year-old child. He excels in school and does not participate in sports. Jason has few friends and often spends his free time alone, playing the flute, reading or watching television. Jason's dad is a stoic, retired Army officer who sells life insurance and his mother manages a local country club. They are frequently away from home, leaving Jason alone to prepare his own meals. Jason has been brought up with a sense of independence and military discipline.

One day, after falling off his bicycle, Jason limped home, complaining of pain in his right thigh. The only sign of injury was a minor bruise, and his father admonished him to act like a "trooper". Jason learned to hide his pain whenever possible, but it gradually intensified and his limp persisted. Convinced this was no more than attention-seeking behavior, his father became less tolerant and arguments ensued. Three weeks passed and Jason's report card was shockingly poor, which only increased family tension.

One morning, Jason's mother received a phone call from the school's principal. Jason had fallen down a flight of stairs and had been taken to a local hospital. She arrived there as her husband was getting out of the car. They were met by the chief of Orthopedic Surgery who stated with remorse that a break had occurred--in the area of a destructive bone tumor. Jason never cried.

Some individuals are conditioned from the start to suppress any expression of pain. Others are programmed to immediately seek medical care or to avoid it until absolutely necessary. Expectations for improvement are often the product of those with whom we live. It is clear that upbringing, environment, friends, associates and health care providers play a major role in programming our pain behavior. Our reactions to pain are based on circumstances, pressures, beliefs, interactions and misunderstandings. From the earliest recognition of pain through our most complex trials and tribulations, pain behavior evolves and develops as perhaps the most primordial yet complex defense mechanism against the dangers of life itself.

Chronic pain has the potential to consume us. It is not surprising that the chronic pain sufferer does not readily have the power to separate, justify or describe what is occurring. The intertwining of self with pain evolves into a maze with poorly defined beginnings or endings. Self and pain grow together and become one, steered though the murky waters of life by our "Invisible Navigator," the mind.

Chapter 4

The Body's Role

Programming by Movement

We are programmed with a set of instructions to avoid movement in order to alleviate pain. It is deeply ingrained that for self preservation, pain is to be avoided at all cost. To worsen matters, our innate fear of pain most certainly reinforces that contention automatically.

Most of us openly accept the concept that the mind has the potential to program the body. However, the reverse is also true, although our awareness of this association is most certainly limited. Understanding and utilizing the concept that the body has the potential to program the mind can facilitate recovery for an individual suffering from chronic pain.

Learning to Listen To Your Body

When a bird breaks a wing, a simple repair using tape to form a splint allows the fragile bones to mend. At some point in time, the makeshift cast is removed and the bird instinctively flaps its wings and seeks freedom.

Human bones must heal as well, and the practice of immobilization is certainly based upon logical scientific principles. Yet to a person in pain, after removal of a splint or cast, the limb does not instinctively move. The brain receives messages from the stiff body part that motion produces pain. Ongoing stabilization, rather than progressive movement, is likely to ensue. The body-mind link creates obstacles that must be overcome to facilitate the healing process. This requires far more than just bone fusion. Fortunately, encouragement, reassurance and structured rehabilitation is often enlisted to stimulate movement, reestablish normalcy and reprogram the body-mind circuit.

At times, we are taught to ignore our body's messages, which leads to detrimental consequences. Football players are programmed to mentally block their body's pain messages. Tackle after tackle, fracture after fracture, these professional athletes continue to pound their bodies irreparably. When they are no longer capable of fighting pain and after ignoring all bodily warnings to stop, drugs or steroids are employed to block the truth. Pain for these players is not a programmed indicator to quit, despite the fact that the aftermath is a predictable life of day to day suffering in a broken body. Programming for these athletes places eventual quality of living as a low priority.

In contrast, as we age, we often tend to become exceedingly more cautious from a movement perspective. If you've never watched a young child learn to ski, you're missing one of life's great lessons. After a few simple lessons, the skis become an extension of the young one's legs. Poles are not utilized as the child does not have a reason to carry extra baggage. Inhibition does not exist and the daring six-year-old throws himself into the mountain, soaring like Superman and catching every bump possible in order to become airborne. Each motion is loose, flowing, rhythmic and free, while sheer delight and excitement sets the quick pace. Falling is just part of the game and no risk is too great. Skiing is fun and exciting!

Contrast the child's experience with the average 40-year-old who manages to break away to the slopes a few times each winter to master the slopes. Imagine the executive who works out at the local spa three times a week to build muscles, increase strength and maintain a healthy level of fitness. Let's follow him through a not-so-unique skiing experience.

During the lift ride to the summit, he recounts his hard work on the exercise machines to give him confidence for the challenge ahead, as he attempts to block out the week's job related stress. After all, skiing is destined to be his release. He gets off the lift, stares down the hill, checks his bindings one last time and deliberately begins his descent. Then, reality strikes! His balance is surprisingly unnatural, even though he spends a major portion of his life walking on two feet. Our subject would not even consider taking on the slopes without his racy ski poles, which he is now using as high-tech crutches. Each movement is stiff and tentative and every spa-tightened muscle is strained to the limit to combat the slope. Our skier's timing is awkward and his rhythm is off. Conscious directives send rapid-fire signals to an obstinate brain, as his eyes are constantly focused to avoid any irregularity on the mountain's surface that could result in a fall. Soreness limits the pace. The terrain is battled constantly in order to descend safely. Getting down the mountain in one piece and returning to the job on Monday, without his co-workers signing a dreaded cast and saying "I told you so," is the brain's primary message. The worst part of this escapade is the fact that our 40-year-old novice is supposed to be having fun!

The child skier is loose and free of worry and concern. His body delightfully interacts with the terrain and eagerly awaits the surprise of each irregularity. His brain welcomes these signals without the slightest reservation and adds colorful imagination to every action. Bumps (or moguls) are exciting and the tougher the better. After all, being a super-hero is awesome!

The adult reads his body's messages differently. Each bump or irregularity is anticipated as a threat. An already sore and tense body sends danger signals to the brain, which tempers these messages with a shroud of fear. This body-mind alliance results in increasing muscle tension in order to counter the hill and survive. Our adult novice's subconscious associations are totally absorbed with self-preservation. Letting go and allowing each muscle to flow and gracefully respond to the hill, using the terrain and gravity to facilitate motion is impossible! The adult skier fabricates a mental body cast in order to avoid pain. He has been programmed to do so. After all, staying in shape is often promoted as increasing muscle tone or bulk. Unfortunately for the skier, this may lead to no more than restricted fluidity of motion.

Pain sufferers respond in precisely the same fashion. The terrain of life is bumpy and each deviation or unanticipated change is dealt with in a fearful or splinted posture. Despite the fact that they claim to relax, these individuals have been programmed by their brain's fear of pain to maintain tension in painful body regions. These sufferers are conditioned to avoid new activities at any cost. The moguls of living become truly insurmountable hurdles. The body's messages to the brain are processed through a fear of failure, not unlike the skier's anticipation of injury or ridicule on Monday morning.

The ability to move is the essence of survival. We often characterize disability in an individual suffering from a painful condition by the degree to which their movement is limited. An alteration in range of motion is considered to be one of the most important objective measures of a pain syndrome.

Our actions and movements program us in a specific manner. The problem, however, is that we are not routinely aware of this essential link. An individual suffering from the acute pain of a neck sprain quickly learns to maintain the affected region in a rigid, non-movable posture, as almost any degree of movement increases pain. Medical care providers reinforce this practice by prescribing cervical collars or similar devices for more substantial stabilization. We are programmed with a set of instructions to avoid movement in order to alleviate pain. It is deeply ingrained that for self preservation, pain should be avoided at any cost. To worsen matters, our innate fear of pain most certainly reinforces that contention automatically. Hence, we are left with a detrimental association; "movement equals pain."

At times, our thought processes are less amenable to change than our affected muscles. We often fail to realize that the maintenance of a static posture (splinting) activates and frequently overburdens a particular set of muscles and inactivates others. If a patient with a neck strain discards a cervical collar after a few days and expands his range of motion progressively through proper exercise, spasm disappears and health resumes. On the other hand, if the patient uses the collar excessively and becomes dependent on it, or if he fails for any reason to reactivate injured muscles, spasm and pain proliferate.

Most healthy individuals consciously expect an unconditioned muscle to become a source of pain when reactivated. Many of us sit in a hot bath, soothing painful muscles and joints after resuming a seasonal sport for the first time in a year. Take a moment to recall how you felt on the first day of tennis or golf after a lazy winter. We accept this pain as a normal occurrence and it does not worry us. Yet, it is often impossible for a chronic pain sufferer to emotionally differentiate the healthy pain of reactivation from the initial suffering of an injury. For that individual, motion suggests pain and pain equals motion. The body-mind link is rigidly established. It's inconceivable to many of us that our brains are actually programmed by our own bodies in an injurious fashion!

In addition to causing pain and spasm, an unused limb or body part can become swollen or edematous after only a short period of time. This fluid build up often results in direct pressure on nerves and small blood vessels, which in turn causes restriction of circulation and further exacerbates pain. The overlying skin can become mottled and any attempt at movement is painful. After prolonged inactivity, muscle wasting or atrophy develops. Bone loss or demineralization occurs as the trophic muscular influence of movement is removed from the skeletal structure. The pain cycle perpetuates itself, as even localized immobility breeds immobility of other body regions. Eventually, the entire person becomes inactive and sick, as the brain is further deceived by the body's messages.

Chronic pain sufferers have difficulty accepting the fact that such substantial physical findings can develop from an improper psychological response to the body's signals. Many people do not consider inactivity as an acceptable culprit for their progressive worsening. The uncovering of a fracture, dislocation, nerve root injury, or even tumor is more palatable to such individuals than anything remotely psychological. To worsen matters further, an improper physical diagnosis can be more believable than the truth.

At times, pain yields abnormal movement patterns that induce and perpetuate suffering. A vicious cycle results and the overall appearance of an individual progressively changes for the worse. Chronic pain sufferers become stooped, rigid, asymmetrical, out of balance and older-looking. They walk less gracefully, take shorter steps and have less fluidity of motion. Restriction of movement sets the stage for diminished activity and pain is displayed with every action

61

and motion. They begin to wear the costume that fits the part! Awareness of normal motion is lost.

Awareness Through Movement

Perhaps one of the greatest contributions to health in our century is the realization that the body can in fact program the mind. Through a lifetime of dedication to humanity, an Israeli physicist by the name of Moshe Feldenkrais proposed a concept that enables people to learn to reprogram themselves in order to emerge from the bondage of pain and disability. The books *Functional Integration* and *Awareness Through Movement* describe approaches to health that clearly delineate the potential to reprogram our existence through the development of practical, logical and natural body motions.

Awareness Through Movement represents a lifetime of Feldenkrais' intuitive, open-minded observation and takes into account the developmental patterns of humans and other mammals. It challenges the accepted alterations of movement that we have erroneously programmed as normal for the aging process. Feldenkrais could identify an inappropriate motion, break it down into components and visualize a more useful one. He was then able to divide that motion into patterns that could be relearned. With a background in the martial arts and a special interest in chronic pain, this physicist-philosopher studied human expressions and proposed detailed lessons designed to retrain the mind through recognition and understanding of the body's signals. Feldenkrais, in his classic book, *Awareness Through Movement* stated:

As soon as we become aware of the means used to organize an expression, we may occasionally discern the stimulus that set it all off. In other words, we recognize the stimulus for an action, or the cause for a response, when we become sufficiently aware of the organization of the muscles of the body for the action concerned.

He clearly believed that the muscles told a story. Whether considering facial expressions or manner of walking, we achieve an important understanding of ourselves through observing and becoming aware of muscular action.

Our muscular activity reflects our emotional life; jubilation, happiness, sorrow, indecision, fear or pain are all manifested this way. A substantial portion of our psychological state is reactive to the messages emerging from our peripheral sensors. Changes in body function are often reflected through complex muscular expressions. In order to understand this seemingly circular phenomenon, we must develop an awareness of what we do to ourselves and how our actions can be modified. Feldenkrais explained this in the following manner:

Movement is the basis for awareness. Most of what goes on within us remains dulled and hidden from us until it reaches the muscles. We know what is happening within us as soon as the muscles of our face, heart, or

63

breathing apparatus organize themselves into patterns, known to us as fear, anxiety, laughter, or any other feeling. Even though only a very short time is required to organize the muscular expression to the internal response or feeling, we all know that it is possible to check one's own laughter before it becomes noticeable to others. Similarly, we can prevent ourselves from giving visible expression to fear and other feelings.

Chronic pain behavior is often expressed as a blend of fear, anxiety and defensiveness. All of these sentiments manifest themselves in clear-cut muscular expressions. I recall a medical school exam that presented simple illustrations of people sitting in a doctor's office, engaged in conversation with a physician. The class was asked to associate a given picture with a psychological state such as fear, anger, apprehension or open-mindedness, by examining the postures and facial expressions of the patients. We all learn to read the muscular expressions of our loved-ones, friends, associates and co-workers. Subconsciously, we use this skill daily to effectively deal with people in our lives. Unfortunately, we often remain unaware of our own expressions.

A person experiencing chronic pain does not notice the tension of his facial muscles, his manner of splinting a hurting muscle or his restriction of body motion in general. Similarly, someone suffering from daily tension headaches is not cognizant of the incessant furrowing of his forehead and habitual stiffening of his neck. Such individuals are not aware that they barely utilize their neck muscles and instead force themselves to rotate their entire body to look to either side. Although the body's messages to the brain sometimes result in restricted activity, "emotions" modulate movement to an equal extent.

Another great student and master of movement and posture, Frederick M. Alexander, a Shakespearean actor from Australia, developed a method for understanding the basis for muscular control of the voice. Through his books, lessons and teachings, Alexander deciphered human motion and used his approach to guide individuals suffering from a variety of disorders. In a wonderful text, *Body Learning*, Michael Gelb, a student of the Alexander Technique, stated:

> My work with the Alexander Technique has helped me become aware of my repertoire of posture and habit and of the associated emotional patterns. I have learnt what I do with myself when I am depressed, afraid, nervous, insincere, happy, attentive and so on. These patterns represent one's character.

Our character cannot be separated from our pain and suffering. Preexisting mental associations often combine with movements to produce patterns of behavior and character traits which can be harmful. At times, such habits limit our potential for recovery and our self-image presents obstacles which may be hidden in the depths of our psyche.

Sadie's Story

A legal secretary for a well established firm, Sadie is an active 64-year-old grandmother who enjoys tennis and square dancing. She and her husband of 35 years, a retired executive, travel frequently, camp out, hike and photograph wildlife. On their last trek through Yosemite in early summer, Sadie slipped, fell six feet, landed on an embankment and was life-flighted to a local hospital. X-rays revealed a left hip fracture and the following day, she underwent a surgical repair. On the third day after surgery, a blood clot developed in her calf, prompting the doctors to prescribe a blood thinner to prevent further clots. Her physician explained that the medication would be needed for the next six months and that another fall or injury could possibly result in severe bleeding.

Prior to discharge, Sadie received physical therapy and was given a set of instructions for limited and safe structured activities for the next few weeks. A follow up with her surgeon prompted a referral to an outpatient physical therapy center for range-of-motion exercises and conditioning. She continued to experience more pain in her hip than she had anticipated, and recovery was slower than expected.

Sadie followed up with her doctor six weeks later and expressed her frustration with the pain and weakness that were preventing her from enjoying the summer's opportunities for adventure. Her physician explained that old bones take longer to heal and stated confidently that she was doing well for a woman her age. Sadie returned home, walked into her bedroom, closed the door and stared at her image in the mirror.

By autumn, Sadie's progress was at a halt and this once vigorous woman fell into a deep depression. Despite the fact that she had been able to walk unassisted to her last medical visit, she surrendered to using a cane as a constant companion. Introverted and fearful, her limp worsened, and she developed a hunched posture very much unlike her characteristic fluidity of movement. She carried herself rigidly and appeared to have aged 20 years in just a few months.

Evaluations by several other physicians revealed no new insights and the basis for her disability was always diagnosed as arthritis. Frustrated with the quality of her existence, she sought the help of a young orthopedist who referred Sadie to a Feldenkrais practitioner in a neighboring city. He carefully explained to her that this was an alternative method of pain management that had the potential to help reestablish functional mobility. Reluctantly, she made an appointment.

Two weeks later, Sadie and her husband were seated in a small waiting room, anticipating another failure. A middle-aged woman greeted them and explained that she was a physical therapist who had been recently certified (after four years of additional training) in the Feldenkrais Technique. Her office contained no complex diagnostic or therapeutic machinery and the exam room was furnished with just a cot and a stool. After briefly describing the Feldenkrais method, the therapist conducted an extensive review of Sadie's medical history, focusing primarily on her activities prior to the injury. An unusual exam followed the consultation. The therapist primarily observed Sadie's manner of lying down, sitting, standing and walking. A gentle hands-on exploration revealed tension of the pelvic musculature, associated with a marked imbalance of muscular forces in the lumbo-sacral or low back regions.

The diagnosis presented and discussed centered on a theory of muscular imbalance and postural instability, coupled with desynchronized and inefficient gait. The therapist told Sadie that she walked like an elderly cripple and that such a costume was not hers to wear. In a caring manner, she explained that Sadie's pain programmed a response that was limiting her potential for recovery. A therapeutic regimen of Functional Integration "lessons" (not treatments) was recommended.

Through several Feldenkrais "awareness" sessions, a frail and rigid specimen of suffering learned to understand her body's responsiveness in order to regain fluid motion. Sadie became progressively more cognizant of "how" she moved and "how" her motions induced disability. After two months of relearning the most basic concepts of walking and reintegrating pelvic motion, her will to live returned with a vengeance. It was a phenomenal metamorphosis of a human being. Sadie recounted these events as her "near death experience" one evening six months later, as she prepared to photograph a majestic sunset over Wailea Falls on the island of Kauai.

According to Feldenkrais, "Death is the absence of movement." Life is motion and to a great extent, the quality of our existence parallels our muscular expression. Sadie was deleteriously programmed to accept a disability, which for her was a death sentence. She was left with a dim prognosis, as a number of well-intentioned medical practitioners were in agreement and accepted her progress as adequate and customary for her age group. Lack of confidence in

68

in the recovery potential of older people prompted a waste-basket diagnosis of "arthritis," rather than a quest for a cure. Sadie's expression of pain, coupled with her submission to the fate of old age, set the stage for a hunched-over, limping, rigid, short-stepped posture. Pain and fear were finally transformed into disability, aging and an anticipation of death.

Society acknowledges that pain and dysfunction are an inevitable part of aging. Fortunately, the concept has been challenged. Thomas Hanna, Ph.D., the director of the first Feldenkrais training course in the United States, wrote:

> No advice is more treacherous than this: Now that you're getting older, you ought to slow down a bit. This is a pathway leading directly to decrepitude. Such advice is not only debilitating; it is deadly.

We have been taught to approach growing older with trepidation, believing that with the advancement of time our bodies naturally become slow, stiff and painful, as the posture of old age sets in. Aging is a natural process, and we should approach it with great pride and satisfaction. We must reeducate ourselves and dismiss the myths of old age.

Sensory Deception

As described in Chapter 2, one may compare the brain to a sophisticated computer that depends on appropriate signals and messages from the outside world to function adequately. We are endowed with a network of external receptors that are vital links with our environment. These signals provide the conditioning stimuli for the development of responses needed for action and survival. At times, however, our sensory apparatus deceives us.

This form of sensory deception is best represented by the story of an Olympic high jumper who trained extensively to improve his technique and set a new world record. His body had been finely tuned to use every muscular action as efficiently as possible to perform his outstanding feats. Yet despite advanced coaching, a focused attitude and incredible perseverance, he could not break the record. Finally, his coach tried a new approach. In a routine practice session, he set the bar at a level which surpassed the existing height of the world record. He told the athlete, however, that the bar was set at a lower point, well within the reach of his routinely successful jumps. The height differential between the two levels was not discernible visually and our subject's perception did not conflict with the information he was given. Not surprisingly, the record was immediately broken. It was accomplished, not by utilizing muscles in a new manner, or by changing the desire to accomplish the feat, but by deceiving the brain with erroneous data. The athlete accepted the challenge as well within normal grasp and success became a matter of fact, as the muscles responded in synergy without inhibition. It is important to realize that this example does not demonstrate a change in attitude or self-confidence. The athlete broke the world record simply because he unquestionably accepted the data forwarded to his brain by a set of peripheral sensors, his eyes. He was visually tricked into believing that the height of the bar was well within his reach. How easily we are deceived!

Programmed Inhibition

As previously stated, human survival is based to a significant degree on primordial instincts and learning. At times, our basic set of programmed instructions seems to get in the way, preventing the learning of new skills and the process of recovery. Our peripheral sensors are constantly vigilant, providing a security network to maintain safety for us. Defensive postures are based upon a flexion and tightening response, sometimes referred to as cringing. This action, which consists of bending the spine, drawing the extremities toward the midline and tucking the chin inward, serves to protect the vital organs in times of perceived danger. Sudden fear elicits cringing immediately, while chronic pain and stress promote the gradual development of this posture. Let's take a few moments to review one of my personal learning experiences.

Skating On Thin Ice

Several years ago, my children began to take ice skating lessons. In order to support their interests and spend some valuable time with them, I decided to try it myself. Not having skated since my teens, at first I was lucky just to circle the rink without falling, holding onto the rail of course. Within a few weeks, despite two very achy feet, I began to feel more comfortable and was actually enjoying the experience. One day, in a fleeting moment of bravery, I decided to attempt skating backwards, a simple feat I had never mastered as a child. I felt confident that, as a neurologist, I could mentally break down the necessary muscular actions and utilize a logical and analytical approach for learning this new skill. Convincing myself that I would have an advantage as an organized and disciplined adult, I decided to further guarantee my success by taking a few lessons. Unfortunately, the experience did not proceed as planned.

Despite a positive attitude, a type "A" unrelenting personality, and a rather scientific approach, skating backwards was an impossible feat for me. I observed many children, studied slow motion videos and even asked my daughter to push me backwards as she skated effortlessly through the arena. Although I fell infrequently, I tripped almost constantly. To state that I felt like a fool would be a gross understatement.

Finally, I watched myself closely on one of our most hilarious home videos. I was cringing. Leaning forward with the cervical and lumbar regions flexed, pelvis contracted and knees bent, the awkward nature of my posture was unmistakably an expression of my fear of falling. One could barely expect to skate forward in that position, let alone backwards. Yet, even after realizing that fear was inhibiting my actions, I could do nothing to overcome it.

When I was on the ice, every subconscious movement was protective, and my own central nervous system would not follow even the most simple command. My conscious mind could not control my body! Every time I took a deep breath, extended my spine and relaxed my legs, gravity set in and all of my proprioceptive sensors lit up like a neon sign and signalled my central nervous system that falling was imminent. In response, of course, I immediately resumed my awkward, defensive posture. Frustration ensued and worsened matters as I observed an entourage of six-year-old children effortlessly skating backwards, giggling at Lauren's dad.

Reprogramming my nervous system was a nightmare. All attempts and approaches failed, until one day I tried a new tactic. I fought to allow myself to fall, proving that the trauma was tolerable. Accepting the prospects of pain, I leaned backwards and carefully positioned myself to follow my instructor's suggestions. I fell again and again and within two weeks my right forearm was swollen and black and blue. I bought a set of elbow pads to soften the blows which somehow became progressively less frequent. Fortunately, I was never injured seriously. I did finally prove to myself that I could lean backward, defy the laws of gravity and suppress all of the inhibition that stood in the way of successfully propelling an obstinate and aching body backwards.

Now, even when stepping onto the ice for the first session of the season, I subconsciously turn around and skate backwards in a fully relaxed and somewhat graceful posture. This activity is so deeply programmed that, like riding a bicycle, my muscles have never forgotten how to accomplish an action which now occurs naturally and without the slightest mental directive. These new connections in my central nervous system are here to stay.

I recount this experience frequently when taking care of patients experiencing chronic pain. I can personally relate to the fact that they are fearful of pain and are avoiding any action that could potentially produce further injury. With the understanding that they are initially not in control of themselves, I anticipate their fear of physical therapy or exercise and attempt to gently reprogram the deeply ingrained association between movement and pain. In order to enhance early progress, our Center's Feldenkrais practitioner teaches muscle awareness prior to embarking on an exercise regimen.

The mind/body alliance is inseparable. For survival, we rely on signals from the brain, which at times cause inhibition and block recovery. Similarly, many of the body's messages program the brain to respond in a manner that initially may be protective, yet later become detrimental to recovery. Reeducation and awareness are key elements for successful pain control. Improving range of motion and reestablishing normalcy of movement often parallels reduction of pain.

Chapter 5

Modern Conditioning

Programming by the Media

Fads do not appear spontaneously; they are specifically programmed. Corporations strategically assemble multifaceted, professional teams and endow them with phenomenal budgets in order to develop an array of advertisements that sway millions of people in a desired direction.

Pain behavior is not purely instinctual. Human action is the product of heredity and learning. Despite the fact that our basic genetic code is firmly established, our expressions are constantly malleable. This feature of life ensures the potential for the learning or programming of behaviors beyond the limits set forth by our basic instinctual patterns. As discussed in prior chapters, internal and external influences serve to shape us and mold patterns of pleasure and suffering. In order to understand the external contributing factors for our actions or feelings, we must begin to study our outside influences. In this society, none is more omnipresent, powerful and potentially destructive than the media.

Far-Reaching Impact

A multibillion dollar media industry, which has evolved to enormous proportions, directs the focus of global learning, utilizing advanced communications technology. We accept this phenomenal network as a fundamental part of our lives, and it transcends practically all physical boundaries. Activities such as watching television, listening to the radio and reading a newspaper are routine in our society.

We often begin the day reading the newspaper with our first cup of coffee. For most of us traveling to work, the radio is a welcomed companion. We watch television as a primary source of entertainment and as a means of staying in touch with a fast paced world. Despite an aggressive, logarithmically expanding cable network industry, there never seems to be an adequate number of television channels. In order to expand our entertainment horizons, satellite systems are purchased to add to the number of available selections. Through advertising, giant industries foot the bill for this universal network. As individuals, we often pay dearly for the link between corporate financial profitability and the media.

The fact that there is at least one television in 97.1 million American homes, and the average American family watches television 47.55 hours per week (according to Nielsen Media Research, 1992) is mind boggling. Most individuals spend more time in contact with the media than with family, friends, hobbies or even work related activities. Between television, radio, newspapers and magazines, we undergo a constant bombardment by unsolicited external influences that support and modulate our major entertainment systems.

The enormity of such a captive audience is frightening when considering the overall potential impact on our lives. When we realize that the underlying basis for commercial advertisements and many programs is the capacity for monetary gain, the content of the programming messages that shape our lives must be questioned. From products used to wash our floors, to the toys which help shape the development of our children, to the manner in which we deal with pain, the spectrum of topics covered by the television industry alone exceeds reasonable limits. Take a moment to conceptually couple the audience size with the repetitive nature of advertising and you will begin to understand the true power of such an organized effort. The magnitude of this influence is further enhanced by subtle, hypnotic, advertising messages that progressively seeps into our subconscious and programs us in a deleterious fashion.

Advertising campaigns are designed exclusively to sell products. To convince the public to purchase an item, ads must induce an alteration of belief that typically results in a change of behavior. The psychology upon which the most successful ads are developed focuses on specific motivational elements, which become deeply ingrained and represent sensitive sources of potential manipulation.

The field of advertising is a well developed and highly supported science. Vast organizations study the human response in detail and viewers' opinions are constantly polled.

Preferences for products are studied and subdisciplines within advertising agencies evolve to characterize and predict reactions to specific forms of external conditioning. Media agencies test the waters through immediate feedback from the manufacturer. As long as a campaign translates into desired sales, it continues to be presented. When a fall-off occurs, a new strategy is immediately summoned into action. This approach is logical, scientific and extremely successful. Fads do not appear spontaneously; they are specifically programmed! Corporations strategically assemble multifaceted, professional teams and endow them with phenomenal budgets in order to develop an array of advertisements that sway millions of people in a desired direction. A successful campaign for a widely used product may result in revenues that exceed the gross national product of some countries!

Linking Emotions to Actions

As discussed extensively in a wonderful tape series, *Personal Power* by Anthony Robbins, man is primarily motivated through seeking pleasure or avoiding pain. Robbins, in an intuitive and analytical manner, suggests that the quest for pleasure is one of the most significant guiding forces in life, yet the avoidance of pain, at almost any cost, is the dominant determinant of our activities. He meticulously describes a credit card commercial that proceeds something like this: An attractive couple in their fifties, upon beginning their vacation, is stranded in Europe, realizing that their luggage has been lost. Within seconds, a programmed response of deep remorse and pain develops for the viewer.

One associates growing old, retiring and saving hard earned dollars for a vacation with an unfortunate, depressing and painful climax, represented by being stranded in a foreign country without resources. Then, almost magically, a credit card appears. The woman frolics through the streets shopping for a new wardrobe while her husband hits an incredible drive on a lush green fairway. The couple meets, embraces, literally dances in the streets under the canopy of a majestic sunset and the credit card reappears. The viewer, in a span of 30 seconds, has been hurled into the pits of despair and suddenly rescued by the elation of love and unlimited spending in a romantic setting. The commercial's detail is designed to serve only as a set of programming instructions. The actual content will most likely not be retained in memory. The message however is clearly retained by the viewer. Sadness and loss is instantly transformed into joy and happiness--which are firmly attached to a credit card!

Anthony Robbins' example demonstrates a method in which advertising agencies take advantage of our emotions andexperiences. Feelings are manipulated and people are programmed in 30 second blips. Such commercials play repeatedly to unsuspecting subjects and program them to respond in a desired manner. Many individuals suffering from depression or pain do not venture out of their homes for work or social activities on a regular basis. Instead, they rely on television to fill hours of frustration. Their vulnerability is easily exploited.

The underlying intent of commercial messages is often not obvious at first. However, when one takes the time to analyze them carefully, their true meanings surface. Unfortunately, the consumer does not typically scrutinize an advertising campaign. It should not be surprising that in a moment of despair, we reach for the plastic and go shopping. The programmed sequence is effective, simple, and spontaneous. The sensation of pain elicits a credit card response that translates into immediate but short-lived pleasure!

The programmed association leading to happiness abruptly ends with the arrival of the monthly credit card bill when the action and consequence become the responsibility of the consumer. It should not surprise you that the corporate profits derived from a million dollar advertising campaign are astounding.

Associations From the Past

The far-reaching impact of television and radio advertising is truly phenomenal. If we recollect the past, certain ads and jingles remain amazingly fixed in our memory banks. Despite the fact that we process an enormous amount of information on a daily basis, we carry certain trivial associations through our lives as seemingly unnecessary baggage. Although we occasionally forget to pick up a quart of milk on the way home from work, or fail to recall a birthday or an appointment, an array of ridiculous jingles sometimes stays with us forever. Take a few moments to recall ads from the past. You will be amazed that sayings such as "I can't believe I ate the whole thing" or "Relief is just a swallow away" or "..and away go troubles down the drain" come to mind immediately. You may no longer remember the product, yet the message is as distinct as if you heard it yesterday. Some recalled jingles last aired 25 or more years ago!

The fact that our minds store these apparently trivial phrases should trigger a sense of concern. We must ask ourselves why such information becomes fixed in our minds while important data, often necessary for overall well-being, doesn't sink in. Are we truly in control of our mind's gateway? Are these phrases simply catchy jingles, or do they represent well-established external programming commands that determine our actions? The answers are disconcerting.

Let's take a few moments to review one of the ads from the past. It unfolded in the following manner. A rather jovial, overweight and deliberately comical character proceeds to indulge himself at a party in a gluttonous manner. For approximately half the length of the commercial, he continues to stuff himself, thoroughly enjoying every second of the never-ending feast. The view then cuts to a scene in his bathroom and opens with our character experiencing sickening indigestion and nausea. He looks in the mirror and moans, "I can't believe I ate the whole thing!" His loving spouse suddenly appears and hands him two pills, which he swallows with an overwhelming sigh of incredible relief. The commercial ends as our subject lies in bed, kisses his wife, turns over and smiles cheek to cheek.

Although lighthearted and almost hilarious on the surface, the message is clear. This commercial insinuates that one need not worry about "pigging out" in order to attain pleasure even though such action might eventually produce pain. When the suffering begins, a few simple pills will immediately remedy the situation. One is simply exonerated for improper and potentially destructive behavior. This lackadaisical approach to health has been programmed deeply into the minds of millions of viewers who are unaware of the basis for their behavior. When we consider this commercial along with similar contemporary ads, our nation's unhealthy eating practices are not surprising.

Although the scenarios of medication ads vary, the messages do not. A company cannot sell a drug to settle one's stomach if it programs the public to eat judiciously. The fact that these campaigns do not encourage preventative or health maintenance practices comes as no surprise. With the exception of commercials for weight loss centers, advertisements do not concentrate on well-balanced meals eaten in moderation. In fact, we're often programmed to indulge ourselves beyond rational limits, only to be salvaged by that which we are programmed to expect--the quick and painless cure. This concept produces irrational expectations and detrimental response patterns.

The Instant Cure

Perhaps the most difficult and frustrating obstacle to overcome in attempting to break through to a patient in chronic pain is the ingrained concept that an immediate cure must exist. People often doctor shop in order to find the one practitioner with the instant cure, whether it be in the bottle or on the operating table. We are not programmed to work through a sometimes lengthy process of healing and are certainly not encouraged to learn about ourselves. Unrealistic expectations often transform into despair and overt frustration.

Health practitioners who treat chronic pain patients are often frustrated with commercials that advocate and glorify the instant cure. A particular advertisement for a pain remedy instills the belief that we are not completely responsible for our own expectations and behaviors. This campaign deserves an award for serving as the classic exemplification of such programming. The vignette begins with a close-up view of a popular, handsome, and rugged-looking actor, who looks you straight in the eye and states, "When you have a headache, bang it back!" The camera zooms to a bottle of popular pain pills and pans back to the smiling actor's face. The message is clear.

We are not instructed to rationalize the basis for pain, to explore its causes or even to seek some form of medical help. Instead, this company has decided to suggest attacking pain head-on with the fury of "banging it back." Although illogical when we consider the script, the programming intent is most effective and the directive is straightforward. Bang your headache back using a drug associated with a well recognized role model to take command of the situation and force the instant cure.

This message is stereotypic of ads for pain medicines. The "pain-pill" connection is so widespread that it has become as automatic as the associations "red-stop, green-go." This form of programming extends beyond the realm of pain into the general medical arena. Advertising campaigns developed for symptoms such as coughing, sneezing, itching, insomnia, and indigestion are commonplace. The same directives are repeated again and again. If you sneeze, take a pill; if you itch, take a pill; if you cannot sleep, take a pill. If you experience a symptom, take a drug! Without doubt, the over-the-counter drug industry is flourishing.

Over-the-Counter Programming

It's important to spend a few moments reviewing the concept of over-the-counter remedies. Years ago it was commonplace for people to walk into a local drug store and ask the pharmacist for symptomatic treatments. For the purpose of our discussion, let's assume our subject had a headache. After a few questions, the pharmacist would reach behind the counter (hence, "over-the-counter") and sell the customer a bottle of pills, with advice to see a physician if the symptoms did not clear in a matter of a few days. Three days later, the sufferer would return, having used all the pills in the bottle. The pharmacist would recall giving the customer medication earlier that week and therefore would not provide another remedy. He would proceed to suggest that the individual visit the family doctor. The approach in a simpler era was certainly a practical one.

Today, nonprescription items are no longer over or behind the counter. They are "off the shelf." Shelves are stacked with more brands of symptomatic remedies than breakfast cereals in a supermarket. In fact, many pharmacies have independent aisles devoted entirely to just one symptom! According to the National Headache Foundation, "Americans spend $4 billion annually on over-the-counter pain relievers, many of which prove ineffective." Walking through such a store and perusing the inventory is an eye opener. In addition to a variety of promotional materials, the counters are stocked with a selection of symptomatic remedies extensive enough to induce a headache if one does not already have one. The degree of generic redundancy is not immediately apparent to the average consumer as the ingredients are typically listed in small type on the back or sides of the box.

A *Potpourri of Similar Ingredients*

Frequently, pain sufferers arrive at a doctor's office with a list of concurrently used over-the-counter medicines. Unfortunately, the patient, in many instances, does not realize that the very same ingredients are being consumed simultaneously through a variety of brand name products. Although relatively safe in recommended doses, the resultant overdosing of such drugs produces a distressing array of side effects which often worsen the overall syndrome. In the end, the victim, not the symptom, gets "banged back."

To complicate matters further, individuals frequently consume multiple medications in precisely the same chemical category, simultaneously. One of the most popular groups of pain remedies in existence today are the NSAIDs, or nonsteroidal anti-inflammatory agents. Over-the-counter drugs such as Aspirin and Ibuprofen are in this category and should not be used at the sole discretion of the consumer. For the most part, certain NSAIDs have been released as nonprescription drugs in lower dosages than prescribed by physicians. Relative safety and freedom from side-effects is only possible when such medicines are used in accordance with normal prescribing practices. Most people are not aware of the true danger until after a problem surfaces. Excessive use may cause ulcers, generalized bleeding and other serious side effects that can lead to serious illnesses.

When an individual has the opportunity to purchase an unlimited quantity of a specific remedy, major problems arise. One tablet every six hours, a few days per month may produce substantial reduction of pain. However, many individuals, unaware of potential pitfalls, erroneously assume that if one pill is effective, two or three at a time will produce better results. Compound this by multiple pills containing the same drug, taken several times per day on a regular basis, and the results are not surprising.

We should not assume that these unknowing victims represent a class of typical drug abusers. That is certainly not the case. These agents are not prescription controlled, nor are they illicit or illegal. For most individuals, such medicines are not taken to experience a "high" or to induce an escape. Many people simply get caught up in taking pill after pill to alleviate or prevent a host of symptoms. Patients often reveal that they take a pain pill after awakening in order to be able to drive to work. Such an established routine is commonplace. After all, the media does not teach us to deal with pain logically; we are programmed to "bang it back."

Pain Medication May Be Harmful To Your Health

The practice of medication overuse does not just extend to nonprescription items. At a headache seminar last year, I mentioned to an associate that a particular prescription pain drug was tremendously overused by the public. He argued that most people used the drug judiciously. Based on our knowledge of "drug rebound headaches," we agreed that proper usage was typically limited to a few times per month. After the conference, we polled the attendants, while I answered individual questions. At least 60% of the group was found to be using such a drug, or a generic equivalent, on a regular basis. Typical consumption ranged from 30 to 150 pills per month!

Let's focus on the phenomenon of "drug rebound." If one takes certain over-the-counter or prescription medicines on a regular basis, the effect of the drug wears off and the symptoms typically return, often with increasing severity. In the past, researchers and practitioners believed that rebound only occurred with truly excessive medication use. Many now believe that taking just a few of the most popular pain pills every day for a prolonged period, such as a month or more, can induce true rebound. This translates into the fact that daily and often debilitating pain may be frequently induced by the pain remedy itself! The term *Transformed Migraine*, has been coined to describe continuous headaches induced through the daily use of pain medications in an individual who initially suffered only occasional intermittent migraines.

Large drug companies promote the use of medicine for corporate gain and not necessarily for the good of society. As a result, many of the patients we treat are so dependent on prescription or over-the-counter drugs, that hospitalization is often necessary to wean them off these agents in order to establish a pain-free state. Of concern to the chronic pain practitioner is the fact that the sufferer is not victimized by just the media; the medical profession does its part as well. After all, someone must be prescribing vast quantities of pain medications to chronic sufferers. One may argue that patients often secure prescriptions from multiple practitioners. However, this is not always the case. Frequently, a well-intending doctor, in order to control pain, progressively prescribes larger quantities of these agents. A regrettable cycle often ensues.

Programming Emotions

Let's focus our attention for a moment on media programming techniques utilized to sell drugs. Medication commercials often utilize specific key elements, such as a family relationship, to produce an effective campaign. Commercials frequently depict mother carrying soup or tea to a sick loved-one and placing a spoonful of a given preparation in family member's mouth. This powerful programming image firmly attaches family values, love and warmth to specific products. Such advertising campaigns often result in programmed messages of immense emotional depth and effectiveness. The media specifically manipulates these feelings to sell medicines. Their objective is to produce an immediate association of warmth, caring and mother's love with a specific product name. Subconsciously, these feelings are reactivated when we stroll down a pharmacy aisle stacked with a myriad of similar preparations under a variety of names. The fact that a specific brand routinely outsells all others is based upon more than just chance or packaging. Our eyes are drawn to the product that has been repeatedly programmed into our subconscious and attached to specific sentiments. This highly effective promotional technique is not limited to medication advertisements.

It should come as no surprise that the media specifically links emotions to products. Not all promotions draw on our longing for warmth, caring and family values. That slinky, sexy and mysterious woman in dark glasses driving an expensive red European sports car arouses predictable responses that are linked to products ranging from automobiles to soft drinks and from jeans to perfume. A trek to a major department store's perfume section provides an overt example of the art of promotion. A seemingly endless array of counters display elaborate and colorful spreads promoting a variety of fragrances. The packaging for each product is colorful, eye-catching, bright and stimulating. Posters depict attractive women and men lounging in sensual settings while fashionable and heavily made-up sales people offer elaborately packaged samples of different products. The decision to purchase a fragrance is based far less on how it smells than the image it conveys. Sexual stimulation sells!

In a similar manner, although there is nothing particularly sexy about a soft drink, advertisers understand well that repetitive exposure to an arousing image produces a specific response that can be coupled to a brand name. A recent television commercial links an elderly black musician, an entourage of slinky dancers and a two syllable repetitive phrase to a soft drink. The statement is not descriptive of the product, yet the feelings evoked from this extravagant production are definitely and effectively linked to the beverage. The commercial is so captivating that children and adults walk about muttering the phrase, subconsciously strengthening the bond to the product. I even catch myself chanting "uh huh" without realizing it. The advertising agency has succeeded in programming a powerful yet simple association into the minds of millions of consumers. Successful campaigns represent the basis for the phenomenal economic position of many major corporations.

Programming Trust

Another effective advertising ploy, especially for the sale of medication, is to enlist a sense of authority or trust to instill confidence in an item. How many times do we hear the phases, "four out of five doctors recommend..." or "most hospitals use..." to sell a health-related product? The authority figure of the older grey-haired physician wearing a white laboratory coat is certainly presented to provide the consumer with a sense of security and safety. The effect is simple. The doctor's image evokes a sense of confidence, despite the fact that he's not your doctor or, for that matter, even a real physician. The end result is a belief linked to a box of pills.

This false sense of security admonishes a sense of concern or guilt. After consuming half a bottle of a popular pain reliever over the course of 48 hours, questions should logically arise in one's mind. Is this safe? Should I see my doctor? One sometimes looks no further than television. After all, commercials provide simple and direct answers.

Of course it's safe! "Nine out of ten doctors recommend this drug." I don't have to see my doctor. After all, he's likely to prescribe the very same medicine! Our conclusions are very specifically and deeply programmed.

Many of the patients who visit my practice for an initial consultation report the consumption of incredible amounts of over-the-counter preparations. It's not uncommon for an individual experiencing chronic pain to take literally hundreds of pills each month. I often imagine that if people were programmed to use such medicines sparingly and judiciously, the negative economic impact on certain pharmaceutical companies would only be exceeded by the benefits to society.

Programming Images

To a significant extent, media programming also shapes our self-image and sense of personal worth. In order to link a specific feeling with a product, as described previously, specific images are presented to evoke specific responses. Commercial models are stereotypic of what we want to be. Although in real life, people exist in all sizes and shapes, advertising agencies traditionally hire attractive and seductive actors and models whom we typically do not resemble. That "good" feeling associated with a product is tightly linked to the image of the person promoting it. Drinking a specific beverage or driving a popular sports car does little for the reflection we face when we eventually look in the mirror. The constant attempt to mold ourselves into an unrealistic physical image eats away at our self-worth. Unfortunately, we are not always aware of the falsity of media depictions of life.

From the manner in which we deal with pain to our choice of buying a car to the establishment of a self-image, the media certainly plays a substantial role in programming human behavior. Advertising does more than just demonstrate a product, it programs society to respond in a specific manner, using a planned and highly calculated approach. The impact of advertising is frequently detrimental. Selling such products seldom promotes a logical or adequate solution to a problem.

Chronic pain victims, as a group, are often highly vulnerable to external influences. Certain practices such as medication abuse and nonproductive pain behaviors may have deep roots in day to day media exposure. Manipulating an individual's emotional state to increase corporate sales suggests philosophical considerations that extend beyond the reasonable limits of this discussion. Recognizing the depth, power, and widespread nature of the media's influence is only one step in the process of beginning to change or modify our behavior. Once we understand the basis for advertising methods, the appropriateness of the term for individual media segments becomes obvious. We call these creations "programs!"

Chapter 6

Crossing The Line

Personal Reflections

A chronic pain syndrome has specific characteristics. It's more than just a hurting limb, a painful back or an agonizing headache. This syndrome evolves into a way of life, encompassing every aspect of one's existence.

T heoretical information has the potential to serve as the foundation for possible change. Yet, instinctively, we do not generally apply such knowledge personally, since we seldom recognize our own deficits and problem areas. For example, people are not aware of the fact that they are becoming addicted until it is too late. Even when the problem is obvious to everyone else, denial provides a formidable barrier to the truth. The purpose of this chapter is to involve you personally in our quest to determine if you've crossed the line and are being victimized by chronic pain.

It is generally accepted that a chronic pain syndrome is a painful process lasting six months or longer. This definition however has extremely limited value from a personal or even clinical perspective. The precise duration of pain is not as important as its associated characteristics. Chronic pain behavior can often be recognized early and appropriately treated if awareness of its basic elements exists. This chapter will provide a platform for the recognition of the expressions of a chronic pain disorder. We can begin to utilize these insights as a basis for reprogramming ourselves.

A chronic pain syndrome has specific characteristics. It's more than just a hurting limb, a painful back or an agonizing headache. Chronic pain often evolves into a way of life, encompassing every aspect of one's existence. Without needing to consult a medical text, we readily recognize the fact that coworkers, friends and even loved-ones are afflicted. The expressions of chronic pain are obvious in actions and conversations and the impact on daily living reflects the transformation of a life centered around a painful process. The recognition of such a change in others is straightforward, yet the awareness of the process within ourselves is often elusive.

Personal Reflections

Have you personally crossed the line into an existence of chronic pain? How can you recognize this state? Throughout the previous chapters, case histories were presented describing many sufferers with explanations of how they were actually programmed. Perhaps you can personally relate to some of these examples.

The key to changing your life successfully is to honestly search yourself. This approach may seem uncomfortable at first, yet important revelations are bound to develop quickly if you follow a few basic steps. Although a life of chronic pain is complex, a heightened understanding, coupled with a logical treatment strategy, can produce wonderful results. Give yourself a chance. Your open-minded cooperation is certainly worth the investment, as so much is at stake. Let's work together to explore certain key issues. We will call this activity your "Personal Reflections Inventory."

Regardless of the nature or intensity of your pain, we must begin by focusing on other matters. We will not even discuss pain for the moment. I assure you that there is a rather important reason for this approach. Choose a quiet time to begin this process. Any time will do, as long as you're unchallenged by other activities or interruptions. Find a few blank sheets of paper and a pen, close your eyes, and relax. Take a few deep breaths and focus on your breathing. Your state of mind is important. Regardless of the nature of any question, answer it to the best of your ability--carefully and honestly. Don't pressure yourself, but, in the same vein, don't put this off. You have to start somewhere, and now is as good a time as any. Answering the following questions can be accomplished in more than one sitting, so don't rush. This is your personal inventory and no one need review your answers. Its purpose is to provide you with an overview of your life.

Certain key elements that may become apparent can help provide direction and insight for your process of learning to reprogram pain. This is not a psychological game. It is the first step on the path to living pain-free. Let's begin to work toward this goal together.

Assessment #1

List five previously enjoyed recreational activities of considerable personal importance that you can no longer perform due to pain. Do not list endeavors related to employment. Your list should include activities that you routinely enjoyed in the past. Be careful not to list sports such as skiing if you attempted this only a few times in your life. The purpose of this question is to uncover true losses from your present existence. With each answer, provide an explanation of why you can no longer enjoy the activity. Is it painful? Are you afraid of injuring yourself? Did your doctor advise you not to do it? Close your eyes and open your mind. Your answers are extremely important. Spend time reviewing your life before pain set in and think about how you felt. If you cannot come up with anything now, relax, put down the paper, and try again later. If you cannot list five activities, place a star after the unanswered numbers. This will ensure that no component will be left blank unintentionally.

Assessment #2

List five important work activities that you can no longer perform. Limit the list to tasks that were part of your job or provided financial benefit for you or your family in the past. Next to each activity, include a short explanation of what in particular is impeding the action. Does the activity produce pain? Is your employer uncomfortable allowing you to perform that task? Are you following your doctor's advice? Carefully sift through the reasons that come to mind. The answers may not be obvious at first. You may list more than one reason for each response. Again, rather than leaving unintentional blanks, place a star near the unanswered numbers.

Assessment #3

List five routine activities you still perform at least three or more times a week. Note any associated problems, and explain how you make your way around them. Do not include items such as eating, dressing or taking care of personal hygiene, for they are too basic for this discussion. Be honest with yourself. These are routine activities that you engage in at least three or more times per week. Don't rush yourself, this "Personal Reflections Inventory" can be completed in several sittings. The quality of your responses is extremely important. If you reach a standstill, you may ask a loved-one or friend for help.

Assessment #4

List five areas of frustration you experience on a regular basis since you began to suffer from pain. Be practical, and don't list responses such as "not being a millionaire" if that was not realistic previously. Search your soul and survey your deepest feelings. Touch base with yourself. Again, this is a private matter, for your perusal only. You need answer only to yourself. Please be certain to list only the frustrations that have developed *since* the beginning of your pain syndrome.

Assessment #5

List five frustrations you continue to experience that started *prior* to the onset of pain. Think back over the years and try to cover a multitude of areas ranging from personal issues to finances, relationships and unfortunate occurrences. Do not list issues that you have effectively resolved. Mention only ongoing sources of frustration. How do they truly impact your life? These answers are critical to an in-depth understanding of yourself.

Assessment #6

This question calls for the development of two lists. Begin by naming your present prescription medications and note the quantities of each taken over the last month. If you are unsure, check the medicine container that provides the name of the drug, the date prescribed, and the original number of pills in the bottle. Also include the prescribing physician's name. Please be certain that your list includes pills you might have used that were originally prescribed for someone else. Next, list your nonprescription or over-the-counter medicines and the respective quantities of each taken in a month. Please also describe how you decide to take a drug at a specific time. Is it prescribed every four hours round the clock? Is your drug schedule based on the way you feel? Do you take one drug if the pain is mild and another one if it is severe? What is the effect of each? Does the pain disappear? Does it worsen or rebound three to six hours after taking the last pill? It may be necessary to track your medication usage over the next few days in order to answer these questions more precisely.

Assessment #7

Carefully review your eating habits. Develop a list of the foods you consume at mealtimes and as snacks. Do you prepare meals or do you eat out? Are meals skipped on a routine basis? Do you eat natural foods or "junk food" items? How many cups of coffee, tea or other caffeinated beverages do you drink in a day? Note the latest time of the day you consume these substances. How much weight have you gained or lost since your pain began? Be honest with yourself. Your answers may be eye opening. Just remember, this is a private matter which only you have to face.

Assessment #8

Do you smoke or drink alcoholic beverages? Note the quantities of each on a daily and weekly basis. Present your reasons for the use of each item. This data is most important and you may need to study these habits closely, as the true reasons may be somewhat elusive. Explain how increased pain affects your overall usage and how the substance itself affects your pain. Also note whether or not the habit has increased or decreased since the onset of pain.

Assessment #9

List the doctors or allied health professionals you have consulted for your present condition. Briefly note your impressions of each. Were they sources of understanding or frustration? Jot down whether or not you benefited from the approaches of each health care provider and list the treatments each practitioner prescribed. Don't limit yourself just to medicines. Modalities such as physical therapy, manipulations, massage, relaxation approaches and biofeedback should all be included. Note your response to each of these treatments. Did you practice at home? How long did you follow a specific program? For each item, gauge its success or failure. Don't forget to mention even the worst results. These experiences are of utmost importance.

Assessment #10

This final assessment is extremely important, so take additional time to focus on it. Describe your understanding of the basis for your pain disorder. Is it related to an accident or injury? Try to pinpoint an event or specific incident that may have produced the problem. Include information concerning your personal feelings regarding the cause. You may refer back to information provided by doctors, health care professionals, acquaintances or family members. You may list a variety of possibilities, even if they appear to conflict. Take some additional time to focus on this issue. An understanding of the basis for your problem may be more important than you can imagine. What do you honestly believe to be your chance for recovery? This question must be answered by you alone. Loved-ones and friends cannot assist you in this matter. Only your thoughts count. Imagine for a moment that you're the doctor and your family is asking about your prognosis. Will you recover, progressively worsen or stay the same? Carefully explain your response.

Reflections Revisited

If you have spent the necessary time to search your soul and answer these questions, congratulations are in order. Your cooperation reflects your courage and determination to rid yourself of pain and suffering. Taking the first step is never an easy task and opening your mind to explore your existence is not a simple matter. In any event, if you've followed through with this questionnaire, you've already achieved the first key to success.

Do not review your responses at this time. Put aside your "Personal Reflections Inventory" and take a break for a few days. When you're fresh, review each of your responses prior to reading the following discussions. We'll cover each section together and carefully begin to reprogram your pain.

Discussion #1

Please be sure to review your answers before proceeding further. You may have responded in a variety of manners. Did you list five activities that you can no longer perform due to pain? Failure to note any of these activities may indicate that your life to this extent has not been significantly affected and that your pain has minimal impact on your overall enjoyment of life. If you did list specific activities, consider the possibility that your sensation of pain may be related to the loss of your ability to perform these rather than just the hurting or typical symptoms ascribed to your disorder.

To take this to a higher level, is your pain more than just physical suffering? Does it represent a loss of self-esteem based upon your inability to live life the way you did in the past? Have you given up on those aspects of living that were a prior source of happiness? Have you been programmed to accept emptiness as pain?

As human beings, we hurt on many levels and it's often difficult to analyze our personal feelings. In order to learn to live without chronic pain, you must begin to understand the many aspects of your suffering. The quality of our existence is based on the way in which the scales of pain/suffering versus pleasure/enjoyment are balanced. Pain often mirrors loss--of a friend, a loved-one or even the ability to enjoy or participate in life's activities. To reprogram pain, you must face and resolve these issues in your mind.

The second portion of this question is centered around your reasons for not performing your listed activities. Are you absolutely certain of your inability to perform them? Have you tried recently? Could you find enjoyment by attempting those activities on a more reserved level or limited basis? Has your doctor advised you not to try? Have you discussed this with your health care provider recently?

Most conditions change on an ongoing basis. You may be able to accomplish more than you can imagine. Just because you're stiff with inactivity, beginning an exercise routine or attempting to participate in a sport that you enjoyed in the past might not necessarily produce problems. At times, the act of just resting, lying in bed or being sedentary produces more pain than effectively using muscles. After all, the enjoyment of participation may change your outlook immensely.

Your doctor may have advised you in the past to limit your activities and to rest. These instructions may have been suggested during the acute phase of your pain and in reality this advice may now represent no more than old news. Perhaps your health care provider is unaware that you have not tried to reestablish your prior level of functioning. It's also possible that deep down inside, you believe that activity could lead to re-injury, worsening of pain and irreparable damage. Is this the case? Is fear preventing you from reestablishing the quality existence you once enjoyed?

Did you try to perform an activity in the past, only to note an overall worsening of your condition? Your response this very day might be substantially different! You may be programming yourself to associate previously enjoyed endeavors with increasing pain. Have you considered the fact that under normal circumstances, engaging in a sport or an exercise for the first time in years would predictably cause some degree of stiffness, tightness and muscular aching? In this context, such a result could certainly lead to despair and depression. Take the time to reevaluate your reasons. A fresh approach may provide some wonderful surprises and a host of new opportunities.

Discussion #2

This assessment specifically refers to work activities and only applies if your condition has affected your employment. If this has not changed, you might wish to proceed to the next section. If your potential for employment has changed, let's work together to resolve this issue. Are you unable to perform all or most of the activities required for your job? Are only certain activities limited? Did you conclude that your job was either producing pain or worsening it?

If this assessment applies, you're most likely not working at present or perhaps you're performing only limited activities. Taking this opportunity to break your job down into respective components can help in determining which aspects you can or cannot actually perform. You must ask yourself: Is even limited work preferable to not working at all? Take into account financial considerations, especially if you are the bread winner for your family.

The fact that unemployment benefits and workman's compensation payments do not continue indefinitely may complicate injury recovery and employment decisions. The legal system sometimes interjects issues that affect your overall well-being. For the purpose of this discussion, I am assuming that you're performing this exercise because you truly wish to improve your life without regard for the financial benefits of illness. This subject is an uncomfortable one. From a physician's viewpoint, I am inclined to believe my patients. You should realize however that some degree of dishonesty exists in the system, producing enormous pressures and problems for those who are truly suffering. In any event, you must be true to yourself.

Let's refocus on why you are not working. Is your employer uncooperative or even hostile? Does just the thought of returning to your old job produce headaches or a sickening sensation? Are you not returning to work because of the overall situation and not the pain? Have you contacted your employer or rehabilitation counselor to consider a change in job description? Has your lawyer advised you not to return to work? Most importantly, do you believe that the steps you are taking while unemployed increase your chances of recovery more certainly than returning to some form of gainful employment? Have you been programmed by the system to believe that not returning to work is in your best interest?

Are your activities at home more or less equivalent to your work responsibilities? Perhaps the overall difference is not as significant as you would expect. You might be able to return to some form of light-duty work and feel better than you do now. Two issues are important for this discussion. The first is that not working may be limiting your sense of self-worth and truly worsening your pain. More importantly however, is the possibility that you have been programmed to equate work with pain. This is an unfortunate association that can build upon itself from past experiences, misunderstandings and less-than-optimal employer-employee relationships.

You may be convinced that you are caught in a trap. The thought of working induces pain, yet the consideration of not working adversely lowers self-esteem, resulting in pain. Either way, the programmed response is painful and destructive. It's not uncommon to feel cornered and the stress associated with this situation has the potential to produce a host of debilitating symptoms. I can assure you that developing an awareness of this predicament is a giant step in the right direction.

Discussion #3

This assessment is basically straightforward. If you cannot list five activities that you perform on a regular basis, you must be either seriously disabled or unrealistic. Are you inactive because almost any endeavor worsens pain? Do you limit yourself to an inactive life because you're afraid of causing further damage?

Sometimes, we get caught up in a vicious cycle; inactivity breeds inactivity. We tend to accomplish less and less each day, often unaware of the pattern. Eventually, even getting out of bed or dressing can become a difficult task. These examples certainly represent the extremes, yet are not uncommon for an individual suffering from a chronic pain syndrome.

Doing less and less each day progressively leads to increased soreness and diminished energy with almost any action. Is this preventing you from reestablishing a quality existence? Are you frustrated by looking at the same four walls each day? These feelings are certainly awful. Did you ever stop to think that such feelings often become inseparably intertwined with your perceptions of pain? Eventually, as your life takes a downhill course, you program yourself to link despair with physical injury. It should be obvious by now that pain means more to you than just hurting.

Discussion #4

Frustration is not always destructive. It can signal you that something is wrong and needs to be corrected. On the other hand, if your life is in total disarray and you are not upset, you have cause to worry. We often do not realize that frustration can destroy us if the warning signs are not heeded.

Are you tense and irritated with life in general? Do you have a sick feeling deep inside that overwhelms your will to improve matters? Have you ever stopped to think that frustration may wear the mask of pain? This impostor can be a deceptive foe that is easily conquered if you train yourself to recognize its appearance. Have weeks or months of illness or inactivity programmed you to equate frustration with pain? Is that sick feeling more than just a physical symptom? Could this explain the reason why all prior treatment efforts have failed?

This assessment focuses on the frustrations that began along with your pain disorder. Is this really the case? Did you experience these problems prior to the onset of your pain? Have you linked pain to these frustrations in order to justify them? Perhaps this understanding explains why facing ourselves often hurts!

Discussion #5

Spend some time reviewing how you really felt before the onset of the pain. Sometimes we allow our awareness of prior frustrations and worries to pass from our conscious memory banks. We often assume that all was well prior to an accident or injury and that the first day of our pain experience began with a specific incident. However, previously existing conflicts do have the potential to set the stage for a triggering event to spark a seemingly radical change. Unfortunately, old frustrations are frequently transformed into new ones and we tend to program ourselves to justify these feelings with our pain. It should come as no surprise that people sometimes subconsciously identify a source of blame for their failed marriages, stressed relationships and poor financial states. No greater scapegoat exists than pain.

Take a close look at yourself. Can you truly recall the quality of your life prior to the development of the pain syndrome? Regardless of what conclusions are uncovered, you should learn to recognize frustration as an important barometer of the quality of your existence. You have the power to develop a positive perspective to free yourself from this culprit. As a human being, you've faced many trials and tribulations in your life. Give yourself credit! You would obviously not have reached this point in life without resolving an incredible number of issues. Don't stop trying now!

Why not take a break at this point. These first five questions were the toughest, and I commend you for proceeding this far. I realize that soul-searching can be an exhausting endeavor. In any event, your self-appraisal should be clearer by now. You probably have more than enough food for thought. When you're ready, let's proceed.

Discussion #6

Hopefully, your medication list is not too long. How long should it be? Optimally, you should not have a list at all, but realistically, your medication inventory probably includes more than a few lines. Physicians generally prescribe medication as their first line of approach to the treatment of almost any disorder. Traditionally, that's how we have been programmed. Rarely are non-drug therapies tried first. Typically, only after several drugs are deemed ineffective or produce side effects, does a doctor try other modalities such as biofeedback or physical therapy. For many physicians, these are second order, lower priority treatment endeavors, often enlisted as last ditch efforts.

Patients are typically programmed in the same manner. Many individuals assume that if they leave a doctor's office without a prescription, the visit wasn't worth the cost. Doctors and patients tend to realize such expectations. Hence, it is not uncommon to review a patient's medication history that spans several pages. The combination of drugs and side effects is often amazing!

How long is your list? How many doctor's names are present? Are you taking medicines from more than one physician at the same time? It's not uncommon for a physician not to be aware that another practitioner is prescribing simultaneously. The next time you see your doctor, be sure to give him a list of ALL the medicines you are currently taking.

Are you consuming so much medicine that you're ashamed to use the same pharmacy for all of your prescriptions? Contact your pharmacists and ask for a list of prescriptions you have filled over the past few years. Most pharmacy logs are computerized and printouts are generally available, especially for submission to insurers for reimbursement at the year end. These lists are often quite revealing!

Do you know why you are taking each medicine and what each is supposed to accomplish? Are you aware of which medicines have the potential to produce dependence, addiction, withdrawal, depression and even drug rebound? Are you tired throughout the day? Do you know which drugs are sedating? Perhaps the exhausted feeling you have associated with pain is actually a side effect or the result of drug interactions. The same line of reasoning applies to depression. Some of the calming agents actually worsen depression. Are you constipated and suffering from abdominal pain? Pain medicines, especially narcotics, induce these side effects.

Are you taking additional medications to counter these effects? In migraine patients, certain medicines can induce or worsen nausea and vomiting. Symptoms you have always attributed to a disorder could actually be ascribed to side effects. Consider becoming an informed consumer and don't be afraid to ask questions.

How many over-the-counter remedies do you routinely consume? Two pills, three or more times a day adds up to almost 200 per month! Can you recall the names of the ingredients found in these preparations? Could you be taking the same substance under different brand names at the same time? The answer is undeniably yes. Many patients feel safe taking a total of eight or ten pills per day as long as they believe these are different drugs. After all, the reasonable limits set forth by the manufacturers' recommendations are not exceeded. When I explain that the same ingredient (found in several brands) is being used in phenomenal excess, many patients are astounded!

Your reasons for taking medicine are important as well. How do you decide when to take a "PRN" or "as needed" drug? The answers are sometimes elusive. Is your decision based upon perceiving actual pain or the potential to develop pain? Many individuals program themselves to take a few pills every morning in order to get through the day, regardless of whether or not they feel pain at the time of consumption. Sometimes, we lose sight of why we're actually taking the drug. It happens to all of us, especially when we're stressed.

As an asthmatic, I have carried a pocket inhaler for most of my life. At times, while under pressure, I reach for the device to take a few puffs. Sometimes however, based upon my awareness of this issue, I hesitate before using it. I pause to ask myself if I'm really having difficulty breathing or if I'm just stressed. It should come as no surprise to you that I often have considerable difficulty knowing the difference. Reaching for the inhaler is a programmed response that I must consciously interrupt.

Over the years, our experiences program us to associate pain with stress. In a sense, it's not surprising that pain could induce substantial fear and stress. No one would debate that issue. Unfortunately however, we sometimes mentally link the stress derived from other issues with certain symptoms. For example, when you're pressured to be in two

111

different places at the same time, stress clearly develops. Without realizing why, do you reach for your pain pills? Are you programmed to associate stress with pain even when pain does not exist? Can you separate stress from pain? When I focus on this issue with my patients, their revelations are frequently disconcerting.

Before proceeding to the next issue, it's important to understand that all medicines are not harmful. When prescribed by a practitioner experienced in the treatment of individuals with chronic pain disorders, certain medications can be helpful.

Discussion #7

A wise man once said, "You are what you eat." We often consider this phrase in jest and for most individuals the subject holds little interest. For the chronic pain sufferer, however, nutrition is of utmost importance. We often find that adequate nutrition is lacking and that the body's dietary needs under the stress of a pain disorder are specific. Two issues must be addressed. The first is centered around adequate intake of healthy foods. The second is based on the fact that certain substances can induce or worsen pain. The purpose of this discussion is not to provide a specific diet but rather to review certain common eating habits that have the potential to impede recovery in a chronic pain victim.

Let's begin by focusing on the first issue. Individuals experiencing chronic pain often maintain poor eating habits. Many patients tend to lose their appetites or cannot eat because of abdominal pain resulting from the syndrome itself or medication side effects. At times, a general lack of interest in their overall well-being develops, leading to infrequent meals or the primary consumption of fast food items. It is not uncommon for chronic pain sufferers to experience weight loss or profound weight gain. The latter places a host of undue physical, circulatory, metabolic and biomechanical stresses on an already compromised body.

A friend and respected colleague, Dr. Michael Margolis, M.D., an orthopedist from California, has maintained a long-standing and strong interest in the nutritional aspects of chronic pain management. After studying thousands of individuals, he uncovered the presence of multiple vitamin deficiencies in his patient population. Many other world-renown pain management experts have been led to the same conclusions. I do not want you to erroneously believe that I'm on the soap box to promote the use of vitamins for all people. This is not the case. It is important, however, to become aware of the fact that a person suffering from a chronic pain syndrome cannot possibly expect improvement without adequate nutrition and the correction of dietary deficiencies.

Chronic pain affects one's entire existence and a sense of worthlessness often surfaces. As a result, many individuals cease to prepare meals and frequently awaken to just a cup of coffee. Skipping meals and eating prepared junk food items is often the rule, not the exception. Inactivity and a poor diet can stimulate weight gain coupled with profound changes in metabolism. That occasional look in the mirror tends to worsen one's personal esteem. In an attempt to lose weight, meals are frequently skipped and many people survive almost exclusively on enormous quantities of either coffee or diet caffeinated beverages. Most often, weight loss does not occur and pain substantially worsens.

113

In addition, excessive consumption (more than a few times per day) of caffeinated beverages serves as a stimulant, increasing appetite, promoting weight gain, enhancing anxiety and inducing insomnia. That "sick" feeling, the by-product of too much caffeine, becomes an important and inseparable component of your pain. You may be programming yourself to associate this feeling with pain. Be honest with yourself. Are you capable of separating the two?

To make matters worse, caffeine, not unlike other drugs you might consume, carries with it a very well-documented propensity for rebound and withdrawal symptoms. The physiological effects of large quantities can be devastating.

Caffeine is not the only harmful substance you may be ingesting. Extensive research has led to a better sense of understanding of other pain triggers. Substances with nitrates, tyramines, preservatives, certain cheeses, chocolate, alcohol and a wide variety of other commonly consumed substances have been noted to clearly trigger migraine attacks in certain individuals. Are you caught in a vicious cycle? Has your pain led to poor nutritional habits that directly worsen your suffering? You might consider beginning to resolve this issue by speaking with your physician and asking for a realistic diet. By the way, taper your caffeine intake slowly and you will be in a better position to avoid withdrawal symptoms.

Discussion #8

Tobacco and alcohol are two of the worst precipitants and propagators of pain disorders. To compound matters further, addictions to these substances are sometimes more difficult to conquer than any other component contributing to a painful existence. Numerous articles have been written concerning the adverse effects of their usage.

A research study published recently in a nationally recognized medical journal studied the effects of smoking on back pain patients. The authors concluded that patients who smoked clearly demonstrated a worsened prognosis for recovery with and without surgical procedures. The physiological effects on circulation and muscle metabolism may be more devastating than ever imagined. Without doubt, the presence of such a psychological crutch interferes with other more practical and healthful approaches toward a pain-free existence. In my practice, smoking is frequently a major obstacle and it is often an impossible hurdle for some individuals.

Most people do not realize that tobacco and alcohol are drugs and should be treated as such. If you use these substances, are you aware of their potential effects? Do you drink to drown your suffering, to ease pain or because you cannot stop? Are you aware of the nutritional consequences? You may be depriving yourself of the necessary nutrients or vitamins needed for recovery. Are you aware of the unfortunate interactions with your prescribed and over-the-counter medicines?

You may be programming yourself to accept the effects of these substances as true components of your pain syndrome. Given the highly addictive nature of tobacco and alcohol, it is often difficult to separate your real feelings from those acquired as a result of these toxins. The effects have the potential to permeate your existence and withdrawal is often associated with symptom magnification. I am always pleased with the degree of improvement and personal growth that occurs in my patients after tapering these substances. Yet I am never surprised by the obstinate nature of pain that is commonplace in those who do not stop.

Discussion #9

How many doctors and allied health professionals have you consulted for pain? Is the size of the list and the results of each therapeutic regimen as frustrating as your overall syndrome? Did they take time to listen closely to your explanations and were you open, honest and complete in the presentation of your medical history? Working with a physician, especially when you're stressed, can be a difficult process. At times, failure to communicate effectively can impede progress and lead to a series of misunderstandings. It is important to realize that frustration can occur on both sides of any relationship.

How do you rate your doctor? The answer is not easy. Certainly, credentials and certifications are important and indicate that the doctor has met the necessary requirements to practice in a given field. Personal qualities vary considerably, as doctors are human beings and as such, come in all sizes, shapes and temperaments. Describing and categorizing "bedside manner" is not easy. How do you know if your doctor is right for you? Two interrelated issues must be considered. The first and most important is the level of caring and concern. The second is based upon the many aspects of your physician's approach.

Patients frequently state that a physician, performing an initial consultation, spent only a few minutes reviewing their history, performing a short exam, reading x-ray reports and writing a prescription. They contend that the entire visit lasted no longer than 10 minutes. Angry because they felt like objects on an assembly line, many patients state that they were not even examined, nor was their condition discussed. Leaving the office disgusted and angry, they harbor resentment for the practitioner. Physicians, upon hearing such accusations, often dismiss such complaints as preposterous. They believe that such contentions are based on the patient's perception of what occurred, which was tempered by a sense of personal frustration. Many complaints, however, are truly justifiable. Certain physicians are more inclined than others to see chronic pain patients. Quite often, dissatisfaction evolves when a close, trusting, physician-patient relationship has not been established.

Caring and concern cannot be easily taught in a medical school setting, nor can these attributes or expressions of humanity be standardized. The best pain management physicians I know have a wonderful sense of charisma that is readily apparent to all. They are open-minded and interact closely with their patients, while inspiring them to recover. These health professionals are more than just diagnosticians; they are good listeners and focus their therapeutic endeavors on the entire person, not just a symptom. A sense of security and confidence with a physician can be established from the beginning through a compassionate and empathetic approach. You will have no difficulty recognizing this type of doctor.

At times, however, an individual's attitude can impede even the best efforts of a concerned practitioner. Some patients do not follow their physician's suggestions, even after extensive and caring explanations. Many people in our society have been programmed to expect the instant cure --the miracle pill to end all problems. Recommendations for physical therapy, exercise, dietary management and counseling are sometimes rejected and doctor shopping ensues.

Fortunately, most people are willing to take an active role when a logical treatment course is properly explained. However, this feeling is far from universal and some pain sufferers arrive at their physician's office with a "cure me" attitude. Such a mindset frequently results from prior conditioning and a host of therapeutic failures. Such patients should not be blamed entirely. Our medical system fosters this contention. We are often programmed to receive the "cure" rather than to learn how to accomplish it.

Let's focus on your level of cooperation for a moment. If you attempted to comply with your physician's suggestions, did you cooperate fully? Have you been following instructions regarding medication usage, diet, exercise and therapy? Did you stay in close contact with your doctor or did you miss follow-up appointments or fail to show up for important tests? Your answer to the following question is most important. Have you been entirely honest with your doctor?

The physician-patient relationship is a precious bond. In order to conquer pain, cooperation, honesty and an open-minded approach is necessary. When the physician assumes the role of teacher and the patient that of pupil, both parties learn and grow from their interaction.

Discussion #10

To a considerable extent, your responses to this last assessment may lay the foundation for your present state. You should take time to answer these questions carefully and deliberately. As demonstrated in prior chapters, one's beliefs and understandings set the stage for action. If you are truly unaware of what may have triggered or what presently serves to perpetuate your disorder, you must ask yourself the following questions: Do I truly understand my problem? Was I ever presented with a reasonable explanation for what has happened or for what is occurring? Have I rejected potentially meaningful explanations? Can I utilize my newly acquired knowledge to shed light on my own problem?

If you're seeking help from a new physician, consider taking a copy of your "Personal Reflections Inventory" with you. A caring and concerned doctor would welcome an organized record of your insights, observations and personal feelings that often do not surface when you're in a new clinical setting.

In essence, our final level of inquiry touches the heart of the matter. Ask yourself: Have I been programmed to accept my pain in a detrimental fashion? Is that which I truly believe a barrier to my recovery? Is my fixed line of reasoning promoting my suffering? In other words, are you convinced that you're incurable?

By now, you have had the chance to organize your thoughts regarding our discussion. Please understand that all aspects of this chapter do not pertain to you. Use your "Personal Reflections Inventory" as a mirror of your existence. Re-read your original responses and consider reevaluating and refining your conclusions. New insights can emerge at any time, especially when you learn to open your mind.

Many people spend their lives searching for the one critical, elusive "thing" that will provide the instant cure. The truth is that such a "thing" does not and never will exist. Working your way through a life of pain is a multidimensional process. Your approach and attitude is as important as the goal. Critical to this discussion is the fact that your first step should not be to find a cure. You must approach your pain by first learning to change your mind. Consider a new course of action. Believe in yourself and begin your quest for a pain-free existence by seeking to reprogram your attitude.

Chapter 7

Mind/Body Technology 101

The Owner's Manual

We must accept the body's responses to a wide variety of stresses as clear-cut propagators of a chronic pain disorder. Stressful associations must be reprogrammed and new ones must be developed to reestablish and maintain overall health.

The process of achieving almost any goal in life is undertaken with the initial consideration of three specific elements. The first is to understand where you are at present, the second is to determine where you wish to be and the last, and perhaps most important, is to choose the manner of getting there. The insights from your "Personal Reflections Inventory" in the prior chapter should have given you a reasonable idea of where you are. Your goal is obviously to become pain-free and a logical way of "getting there" is to reprogram pain. This chapter focuses on the psychophysiological, or mind/body link, and serves as a basic instruction manual for reprogramming bodily responses.

The mind/body balance is constantly changing. Despite extensive research, the inherent complexities of this dynamic relationship have not been fully deciphered. The process of developing a comprehensive understanding of this alliance is formidable, and new insights surface each day. We have documented the specific nature of an autonomic response, yet must contend with the fact that a wide variety of stimuli can evoke the very same effect.

The Problem Surfaces

According to the English psychiatrist Henry Maudsley, "The sorrow which has no vent in tears may make other organs weep." This insight describes the plight of the chronic pain sufferer. A host of feelings such as fear, anxiety, stress and frustration induce similar effects including changes in blood pressure and heart rate, constriction of blood flow to certain key regions and increased secretion of gastric acid. Such responsiveness is not stimuli specific. In other words, the feelings that are typically associated with pain are not always evoked by pain itself. We accept certain sensations as characteristic of chronic pain when their origins may be distinct. As a result, we deceive ourselves into developing a picture of pain based on incorrect beliefs. Rarely do we learn to control our body's responses.

Let's consider a simple example demonstrating a system that is out of control. Suppose you invest in a security system for your home. Through a series of motion detectors, it can sense the presence of an intruder and trigger a loud siren and flashing lights. The installer, however, fails to include a switch to disarm the system, once motion has been detected. In effect, your alarm system is *always* on. Every time a member of your household would pass through a protected area, the alarm would sound and the lights would flash. Living in your home would be impossible. Your alarm system would serve no practical purpose if it could not be armed to protect your house when you were away and disarmed at all other times.

Imagine for a moment what would happen if your internal alarm system functioned in more or less the same manner. Your body's protective circuitry would be enabled and vigilant at all times. Pain, stress, anxiety, or almost any stimulus would immediately set it off and the resultant effect, regardless of the stimulus, would be horrendous. Although intended to be a protective circuit, your body's constantly triggered alarm system would eventually destroy the individual it was assigned to protect. In order to survive, you would have to learn to reprogram your alarm system, the autonomic nervous system.

Establishing control of our internal responses is tantamount to recovery. Learning to reprogram potentially detrimental processes can lead to an effective path toward a pain-free existence. Failure to do so results in progressive deterioration of quality of life for many pain sufferers. Most of us are initially skeptical about the prospect of learning to control supposedly automatic body functions. In a similar manner, many people are resistant to believing that pain can be programmed by external influences.

In an excellent paper by Ian Wickram, Ph.D., published in *Professional Psychology: Research and Practice*, applied psycho-physiology is presented in practical clinical terms. He discusses the reticence of certain individuals to accept the possibility that their own physiological response to psychological stress are responsible for their pain. These individuals have been programmed throughout their lives to believe that the diagnosis of illness or pain related to stress is an overt declaration of mental illness and a one-way ticket to a psychiatrist. This serves as a reasonable explanation for the disappointment many people suffer if a clear-cut physical problem, regardless of severity, cannot be uncovered to justify their pain.

Wickram discusses a technique utilized to demonstrate the mind/body relationship to a doubting subject. During an interview with a patient, he places sensors on skin surfaces overlying certain muscles and allows the subject to view the readings. A stable and comfortable baseline is established through a nonthreatening line of questioning that spans a few minutes. The interviewer then questions the leery patient about particularly stressful issues. As the subject responds, the monitoring device reacts to indicate the changes in baseline muscle tension levels. In this manner, the physiological reactions to the anxiety-producing questions become obvious to even the most doubting individual. This "prove it to me" approach produces dramatic changes in personal awareness for many people.

The Missing Link

The term *autonomic* refers to the portion of the nervous system that was once considered a functionally independent entity, typically operating below the level of consciousness to maintain a stable internal environment. The fact that this component of the nervous system was not entirely separate, vegetative or involuntary surfaced in the early 1900s, yet practical training in this area did not evolve until the 1970s.

The autonomic nervous system (ANS) maintains control over many bodily functions. The heart, lungs, blood vessels, digestive, urinary and reproductive apparatus, certain glands and the eyes are affected by this system. To a certain extent, the balance of our entire internal environment is maintained by two components of the ANS, the sympathetic and parasympathetic divisions. These two systems functionally oppose each other in order to maintain a delicate internal balance. For example, the heart speeds up with sympathetic stimulation and slows with parasympathetic influences.

Ancient civilizations recognized mind/body stress responses. Criminals were sometimes judged by a rather unique lie detector test. During interrogation, a pebble was placed in the mouth of the accused and subsequently removed. If the pebble was moist, freedom was in sight. A dry pebble translated into a rather shortened lifespan for the stressed victim. Under those circumstances, diminished anxiety levels did not always mirror the truth. Although the test was not particularly reliable, at least the basic concept was understood!

Despite the fact that ancient texts have described meditational techniques for more than 5,000 years, the clinical practice

125

of psychophysiological self-regulation, termed *biofeedback*, is now entering only its third decade. Once shunned as an impossibility, it is now clearly established through extensive research and clinical studies that voluntary control over many physiological variables is possible. Although termed an "alternative" treatment endeavor by some, biofeedback has received widespread medical acceptance and is presently practiced in most major pain centers throughout the world.

Before proceeding to an explanation of the practice of biofeedback, let's consider the following example. Suppose you are sitting in your living room, reading a book and you are asked to set the temperature of the room to precisely 70 degrees. For the sake of this discussion, the numbers on your thermostat have been erased. The room temperature feels "normal" and in fact, comfortable. You ponder the issue for a moment and readily come to the conclusion that you can not decide whether the actual room temperature is above or below 70 degrees. The dilemma is knowing which way to adjust the thermostat.

Unfortunately, as sick as we may feel, the physiological processes within us are often elusive. Human beings did not evolve with control panels indicating levels of internal function. Changes such as increased blood pressure or muscle tension are rarely discernible. Instead, we feel tense, exhausted and miserable. It's amazing that our body's internal balance can be so disrupted and yet we do not have the slightest clue to where the problem lies.

In order to begin reprogramming pain, we must learn to regulate these functional processes. A valuable tool utilized for this process is biofeedback. The principles of biofeedback are based upon three elements. A specific physiological parameter must be measured with an appropriate apparatus. Typically, muscle tension, skin temperature, skin resistance, pulse, blood pressure or brain wave activity is chosen. The second element is the display of the appropriate measurement or change for the subject. Traditionally, this information is presented as bars, colors, circles or objects that vary according to the body's response. Frequently, these displays are accompanied by sounds or tones that correspond to changing levels. The third and perhaps most important element is the technique used by the biofeedback technician to induce the targeted response.

A biofeedback session for muscular relaxation generally begins by connecting a series of sensors or electrodes to the skin over a preselected muscle. The electrodes are connected via a series of wires to an electronic box that filters out unwanted signals and amplifies the muscle energy in the selected area. Most modern systems utilize a computer to display the signals and keep track of muscular activity during the session. The subject sits in a quiet room and observes the computer screen, while changes in muscle energy are typically converted into moving bars or graphs accompanied by varying tones. The technician directs the subject to alternately tighten and relax a specific muscle, while observing the screen. It soon becomes apparent that the computer display mirrors the subject's responses.

The technician supplies a series of relaxation or induction suggestions and the subject progressively learns to gauge the depth of relaxation by closely following the indicators.

Effective biofeedback, however, is actually based on self-experimentation. The subject moves about, deepens breathing, alters jaw position, opens and closes the eyes and simultaneously observes the effect. Minute changes in posture, for example, can sometimes produce marked reductions in the degree of muscle contraction in a given region, resulting in substantial improvements in pain. The subject eventually fine tunes a relaxation strategy by observing the computer's responses. Through the use of imagery and progressive relaxation techniques, you can learn to lower the levels of muscle tension while reorganizing patterns of movement that were previously destructive and pain inducing.

Of importance is the fact that clinical biofeedback sessions represent only one aspect of overall training. The key to success is clearly related to exercises performed at home or in the work environment that are intended to simulate the feelings derived from the clinical experiences. You are taught to rely on the awareness and sensations experienced during the clinical sessions rather than developing a dependency on the actual biofeedback apparatus. Many individuals begin home exercises by practicing learned techniques in a quiet setting while in bed, prior to sleep. As you become more proficient, exercises are carried out in environments that are progressively more distracting. It is important to realize that effective control over your bodily functions is a skill that must be learned and reinforced with practice.

Biofeedback is used for a wide variety of disorders such as headaches, back pain, Reflex Sympathetic Dystrophy, anxiety, panic disorders and attention deficit disorders. In the field of pain management, we typically enlist electromyographic or muscle biofeedback to attain two specific goals. The first is to enhance the overall relaxation of an individual through the gradual lowering of generalized muscle tension. The second goal is to develop a very specific tool to treat a painful episode. In other words, rather than reaching for a pill at the onset of pain, the subject performs biofeedback exercises to relax certain muscles in order to reestablish a comfortable state. The effects are gratifying and without side effects, as they are achieved naturally.

At times, other types of biofeedback measurements are utilized for pain sufferers. Temperature control has been demonstrated to prevent the development of headaches in classic migraine patients during the warning phase or *aura*. It has also been enlisted as a treatment for an extremely painful disorder which was presented in Chapter 2, Reflex Sympathetic Dystrophy. The electrodermal or sweating response, is also used as a basis for training individuals with similar disorders.

Biofeedback is an integral component of the holistic pain approach. Most of our patients enjoy the sessions and gain self-esteem and confidence by learning to control or prevent the development of pain through non-pharmacological means. It is not uncommon for people with long-standing histories of severe pain or headaches and a profile of drug dependency to develop skills in biofeedback that help to maintain a pain-free, drug-free state. In our Center, Mindscope®, a new and exciting form of biofeedback, represents a quantum leap forward for reprogramming pain. Prior to discussing this technology, let's consider the following scenario.

Programmed Responses

Suppose for a moment that you're in your yard teaching baseball to your eight-year-old child for the first time. After a seemingly endless series of misses, the bat finally connects with the ball and a sense of jubilation and pride immediately abounds, as you smile cheek to cheek. A second or so later, the sound of shattering glass emanates from your neighbor's property, piercing the silence. Instantaneously, a lump in your throat coupled with a deep sense of panic overtakes your exhilaration.

In a matter of seconds, you were dramatically hurled from an all encompassing sense of excitement to the depths of a sickening state. That uncomfortable feeling deep down within prevails as you contemplate facing your less than friendly neighbor. The magnitude of such mood swings in such a short period of time is phenomenal! How can such feelings change so quickly?

The answer is rather straightforward. Specific stimuli evoke both emotional states. Exhilaration and remorse are triggered reflexly and are associated with massive autonomic changes. Observing your child hitting the ball induces a very positive feeling, while the shrill of shattering glass delivers a massive psychological blow. We develop such responses by repetitive programming through our repertoire of life's experiences. We subconsciously recall and differentiate actions that tend to evoke pain or happiness. These experiences program us to react immediately in a specific manner. Our autonomic nervous system has the innate property of almost instantly assuming control, which explains our rather efficient level of responsiveness.

At times, when we are alone and quiet, the pressures of life surface to interrupt even the simplest of pleasures. Human beings tend to ruminate on specific experiences as well as unresolved and uncomfortable issues. Attempts to distract ourselves often fail. Even when we appear to be focused on the task at hand, those worrisome feelings resurface and trigger unfavorable physiological responses without our knowledge. Even the solace of sleep does not provide an escape from the pressures of our life.

The human central nervous system remains constantly vigilant and reacts predictably. Important problems arise, however, when this complex system cannot differentiate a real threat or event from a perceived or even imagined one. Lee Pulos, Ph.D., a world-renowned expert in the fields of psychology and imagery, has described several cases of individuals who have suffered throughout their lives based on adverse conditioning from a solitary event. The critical issue that surfaces in his presentations is that for some of these people, the event never actually occurred! For others, the perception of what had occurred is inconsistent with the actual event. Stop for a moment and imagine how easily we can be deceived! Dr. Pulos introduced the concept that man, under certain circumstances, has the potential to change the past, by reexamining a series of triggering events through hypnotic regression. Associated programmed responses, however, are not easily broken.

Joan Borysenko, Ph.D., cofounder and former director of the Mind/Body Clinic of Harvard Medical School, addresses this issue in her best selling book, *Minding The Body, Mending The Mind*. She states:

> Conditioning is a powerful bridge
> between mind and body, and a primary
> focus for our work at the clinic. The

reason is that the body cannot tell the
difference between events that are actual
threats to survival and events that are
present in thought alone. The mind
spins out endless fantasies of possible
disasters past and future. This tendency to escalate a situation into its
worst possible conclusion is what I call
awfulizing, and it can be a key factor
in tipping the balance toward illness
or health.

Those worrisome thoughts are not independent travel-
ers. We are often overwhelmed by their associated autonomic counterparts that spring into action in a seemingly
uncontrollable fashion. Our worries continue to program
specific and predictable physiological responses, despite the
fact that we attempt to consciously flee from their presence.

Some people succumb to their worries and eventually
resign themselves to lives of misery. Some drown their suffering in alcohol or drugs. Others constantly drive themselves toward external achievement, fleeing from reality and
never finding inner peace. Sometimes, we are afraid just to
stop, take a deep breath, and allow our minds to aimlessly
wander. Uncomfortable reverberations of the past seem to
surface and haunt us. Successful people, however, learn to
focus their minds and reprogram their responses to those
unwanted invaders.

Values, ethical concerns and codes of living are distinct
for each of us, as are our fears and frustrations. Our wor-

ries vary and our perspectives of life are diverse and often change depending on our mood. Yet the overall autonomic response is not unique for the most part. Regardless of the nature of the concern or worry, our ANS predictably reacts in a stereotyped fashion.

When discussing these issues with patients suffering from chronic pain, I attempt to clarify and differentiate a *cause* from a *triggering factor*. The *cause* is explained as the basis for the problem, while the *triggering factor* evokes a response if a specific set of conditions exists. I emphasize the fact that such problems are multifaceted, and I frequently present the following example:

Imagine trying to move an 1,800 pound snowball in my parking lot. We proceed to push as hard as possible, yet it obviously will not budge. Next imagine two skiers, you and I, resting at the peak of a wonderful mountain. We inadvertently lean on a similar snowball which is precariously balanced on a ledge. The snowball breaks loose, causing an avalanche and destroying the chalet at the base of the mountain. The question I ask is: Are we responsible for *causing* the damage? The most frequent response is that we are not. It is obvious that the avalanche was likely to occur anyway as it was only *triggered* by the unsuspecting skiers. A snowstorm, rain, wind or even the thaw of a bright sunny day would have *triggered* the very same response. The damage was actually *caused* by the snowball's position.

As an example, in the case of a migraine sufferer, it is explained that the *cause* may be related to a genetically transmitted biochemical abnormality or malfunctioning neurovascular structure, which establishes the *setup* for the development of headache by a host of *triggers*. Worry, anxiety, or distress induce specific autonomic responses, that have the potential to *trigger* the development of the actual headache. This *setup* has been graphically described by others in terms of a stick of dynamite residing in the head, which can be ignited by a host of potential *triggers*. This linking of a specific worry to a predictable autonomic response may act as a predictable trigger.

For a back pain sufferer, the *cause* is generally explained in terms of an acute injury, a series of traumatic events, or imbalance in muscle forces resulting in muscle, joint, soft tissue or disc involvement. This depends, of course, on the specific case. For a chronic sufferer, the realization that certain *triggers* can perpetuate the syndrome is of utmost importance. When presented in this fashion, many individuals openly relate to the fact that just thinking about their job supervisor or employer increases tightness and worsens their overall suffering. An argument with a family member, a late workman's compensation check or a second payment notice evokes the very same response. Many of us have been programmed to develop similar autonomic responses to stressful issues.

As a physician, I choose to avoid the term *psychosomatic*--not necessarily for the intended meaning but rather for its general connotation. This term is freely used to imply the following: an individual without a clear-cut physical problem, who develops a condition that exists entirely as a result of psychological conflict. For example, this term has been erroneously used to describe the migraine sufferer. It is inconceivable with our present fund of medical knowledge to believe that such syndromes develop on a purely psychological basis.

In a similar manner, the practice of prescribing only a muscle relaxant to reduce chronic muscle tension is equally shortsighted. We must accept the body's responses to a wide variety of stresses as clear-cut propagators of a chronic pain disorder. Such stressful associations must be reprogrammed and new ones must be developed to reestablish and maintain overall health.

The Evolution of Biofeedback Technology

In the mid-1970s, simple biofeedback instruments became available from a limited number of suppliers. The units were rather basic in design and straightforward in operation. The early biofeedback laboratory was built around a series of "black boxes," each designed for a specific parameter such as muscle tension or temperature. The subject typically observed an analog meter (a scale with a moving needle) or a series of lights. Most instruments incorporated a changing beep or tone that varied in volume or frequency as the measured function fluctuated.

The design of such instruments evolved slowly and relatively few technological advancements occurred throughout the early years. In the late 1970s, however, the personal computer surfaced and by the mid-1980s, biofeedback instrumentation developers began to utilize these new devices to display or feed back information to the subject, while recording data for analysis in the background. Many systems today are designed to record and utilize multiple parameters such as muscle tension, skin resistance and temperature simultaneously while recording and analyzing data in a variety of manners. A choice of displays is available and may include graphs as well as changing colors or objects that vary in size or shape.

A few years ago, the opportunity to reevaluate biofeedback in the field of pain management surfaced and many lessons were subsequently learned. Through an avid interest in the field of computing, I approached biofeedback from both clinical and technological perspectives. A careful assessment of the technology led to several interesting conclusions regarding the current biofeedback process.

Many patients learning biofeedback were inherently uncomfortable with the computer. This was especially notable in the elderly or in individuals without prior exposure to or experience with computers. Some people were even "computerphobic." Unfortunately, such apprehension did not necessarily diminish over subsequent sessions and according to several individuals, the technology itself often interfered with their ability to relax.

Lack of continued interest also became apparent. Spending 20 to 30 minutes watching a circle grow larger or smaller was often a difficult task and after a relatively short period, boredom set the stage for a wandering mind coupled with surfacing worries and increasing tension. Many individuals complained of substantial difficulty following a moving bar graph or changing shape for periods longer than a few minutes. Tracking more than one parameter at a time was also disconcerting. Auditory feedback in the form of beeps and tones was considered annoying and distracting for many people. Although some individuals learned to adapt to the technology, the general consensus shed doubts on the overall value for many patients.

Perhaps the most unsettling revelation at the time was the fact that many individuals were not practicing on their own. This was of particular concern in view of my contention that the ultimate goal of biofeedback therapy was to effectively use it in the subject's environment. It was not intended to be just a clinical exercise. Excuses for failure to practice ranged from "not having enough time" to "marked difficulty sitting at home, trying to recreate the biofeedback experience in the midst of all of life's typical pressures." Despite encouragement by our committed staff, it became obvious early on that many individuals did not relate well to the technology.

Even in view of these disconcerting discoveries, I still believed that biofeedback had the potential to play an integral role in the holistic method of treating a chronic pain sufferer. The consideration of advancing biofeedback to a new level prompted the development of Mindscope.®

Mindscope

At the annual American Association for Applied Psychology and Biofeedback meeting in Colorado Springs in March 1992, Mindscope emerged as a blend of philosophy and technology developed to improve the quality of life for millions of people throughout the world.

Mindscope was developed as the first system in the world that utilizes the beauty and reality of nature to teach relaxation through biofeedback in a rather unique manner. Mindscope allows bodily functions such as muscle tension, skin temperature, blood pressure and brain activity to control an incredible audiovisual environment. The patient no longer watches a graph or object change shape on a computer screen or listens to a changing tone while learning relaxation. Instead, utilizing a large screen, high definition television set, subjects watch actual laser video scenes coupled with realistic digital stereo sounds, which are integrated by a completely unobtrusive computer in the background and controlled by the person's physiology. The subject no longer faces the computer.

Mindscope is a new concept based on two straightforward premises. The first is that most people learn best through a realistic audiovisual environment, the foremost of which, in our society, is television. The second premise transcends the boundaries of traditional biofeedback into what we describe as "conditioning." Mindscope provides a wonderful and relaxing scene, the reality of which is controlled by the subject's physiology. The patient is rewarded for developing a deeper state of calm by changes in the audiovisual environment that affect clarity, perspective, motion and sound realism. The scene is used to evoke a conditioned response: a calming, relaxing and tranquil sensation that serves as a very effective treatment for a host of medical disorders.

Shortly after introducing this approach, a patient stopped me to describe an unusual experience. She was delayed in the traffic of a western Pennsylvania snowstorm and was having trouble controlling her car on a rather slippery road. As her anxiety level increased, tension began to develop in her neck and a typical headache ensued. This individual did not reach for a pill, nor did she attempt to perform a relaxation or stretching exercise. She inadvertently blinked her eyes for a second and recalled the image of a white bird peacefully flying across the Mindscope waterfall scene. To her astonishment, the neck pain and headache almost instantly disappeared. She experienced a conditioned response, the true essence of Mindscope.

Initially, 25 headache and pain suffers, undergoing traditional computerized biofeedback training, were surveyed after the performance of a Mindscope biofeedback session at our center. Comparative ratings of traditional and Mindscope sessions revealed the following: subjects indicated that Mindscope enhanced relaxation, produced less distractibility, heightened interest in home practice and promoted an overall sense of comfort and enjoyment to a degree that had not been previously experienced with conventional training. In addition, the respondents noted an increased inclination to continue biofeedback training through the Mindscope protocol. One hundred percent of the subjects indicated a preference for Mindscope over traditional, computerized biofeedback. These positive and enthusiastic responses were based, to a significant degree, on the audiovisual environment, upon which the program was developed. It is not surprising that similar impressions have been noted by individuals in centers throughout the U.S. and in other countries.

Mindscope harnesses the power of television, which is perhaps the most effective communications medium in the world. It is also the most suggestive and comfortable learning technique for most individuals. As stated previously, effective advertising campaigns rely on conditioned responses, and we often choose to purchase a product based on subconscious conditioning. A particular brand of jeans immediately catches our eye as a result of the feeling we experience watching an enticing and seductive character promote the product during a television commercial. This is an incredibly powerful form of conditioning--also a potentially harmful one. Mindscope, however, combines television and conditioning to promote a healthy response.

I often ask people what they do for relaxation. Watching television, playing sports, smoking a cigarette, drinking a beer and playing video games are all common answers. These activities often become associated with harmful physiological responses that are erroneously believed to be relaxing! In effect, I suppose that most conditioned responses are learned unfortunately through stimulation rather than relaxation. Our subjects are taught to develop a very specific learned response, shaped and profiled through Mindscope training and based on a beneficial physiological profile. Overall improvement develops naturally as one learns to reprogram the important aspects of a painful existence.

Over the past few years, our experience with Mindscope in other areas has led to important conclusions. Through a well-controlled study, Mindscope has been shown to substantially improve retention and comprehension in a host of subjects. We have also successfully treated individuals with Attention Deficit Hyperactivity Disorder (ADHD) to improve the overall quality of their lives. It appears that Mindscope's effectiveness is based primarily on the induced receptive state of the user. The key to learning just about any subject or mastering a specific technique may be based, to a significant degree, on successfully establishing an enhanced state of physical calm coupled with a heightened state of interactive mental focus.

Preliminary investigations have also suggested substantial improvements in the levels of circulating neurochemicals and immune modulating substances for subjects undergoing Mindscope sessions. This limited data demonstrates a potentially favorable chemical and immune response. The proper combination of imagery, biofeedback and conditioning through Mindscope represents an important key to reestablishing a state of healthfulness.

The Future

As we advance in medicine and the behavioral sciences, new developments will continue to shape our lives. The study of the mind, perhaps the most exciting frontier in science, will undergo a wholesome evolution. When physicians and allied health professionals learn more about chronic pain as an all-encompassing entity, substantial advances will naturally occur.

For today's pain sufferer, reprogramming one's life must include a comprehensive approach for controlling detrimental physiological responses that worsen suffering and enhance chronicity. Heightened self-awareness is an important key for successfully overcoming a life of chronic pain.

Chapter 8

Convergent Therapy

Synergy In Pain Care

*A cooperative patient, coupled with
a devoted, multidisciplinary team, will
produce results beyond your greatest
expectations. If you accept this challenge
with the goal of reestablishing normalcy in your life, pain can diminish
and eventually disappear.*

The goal of living free of pain is realistically attainable through the process of personal re-programming. Although we have the potential to follow the necessary steps to reach such a goal, the starting point is often elusive. Most often, we do not know where to begin or how to get started. Even when strategy is finally transformed into action, frustration and despair become formidable adversaries that have the potential to undermine even our best efforts.

Each of us maintains a unique set of strengths and weaknesses. The basic problem, however, lies in the fact that we are, for the most part, incapable of recognizing or even characterizing these attributes in ourselves. Therefore, an external and somewhat more objective and critical perspective is often essential to improve our chances of attaining almost any goal. This practical approach for fine tuning even the best of our abilities has been utilized consistently by the world's greatest athletes. For even these brilliant competitors would be unable to achieve their dreams without one essential element--the coach.

Comparing your goals to those of a world class athlete may seem ridiculous at first. If stricken by chronic pain, you probably do not feel even remotely successful from any vantage point. Furthermore, where could you find a coach to guide you to a pain-free existence? The answer is truly within your grasp, as certain medical practitioners have dedicated themselves to this role. The challenge, however, is finding the right coach.

Before embarking on a quest to find such a health care provider, a few very essential elements must be reprogrammed, beginning with your most basic perspectives. From this moment forward, you must no longer seek the "cure." Immediately discard the "cure me" attitude and replace it with a new approach. Dedicate yourself to learning how to cure yourself! Learn to enjoy being the student again. Next, focus on your doctor's mission. The "healer" image must be erased from your memory bank. Reprogram the physician to the position of coach or teacher.

Your understanding of these roles coupled with a reasonable and honest approach can set the stage for a meaningful patient-physician relationship. Such a partnership is essential if you wish to live free of pain. One of the most intuitive scientists of our time, Norman Cousins, once aptly stated " ... the idea of a patient-physician partnership is not just a pretty slogan but a functional necessity and reality." If you allow the physician-patient relationship to evolve into a teacher-student alliance, one will naturally inspire the other.

Bernie Siegel, M.D., in his wonderful book, *Peace, Love and Healing* emphasizes the quality and fulfillment that can develop through a meaningful physician-patient relationship. He states:

> It is when I can help my patients find what Schweitzer called the doctor within - when I play coach, as one of my patients put it - that I am most fulfilled in my role as doctor and I serve my patients best. We become a team with joint participation and responsibility.

How do you set out to find the right practitioner? The answer is not simple, yet by developing reasonable expectations you will become an enlightened and informed consumer. The purpose of this chapter is to provide a framework for a logical and meaningful approach to seeking the very best medical care possible.

It's not surprising that you're frustrated with the medical system. Had it worked in your case, you might be absorbed in a wonderful novel rather than reading this book. Don't ignore your frustrations; take the time to reprogram your disappointments into meaningful energy. Many people living with chronic pain are unhappy with themselves and their physicians. Anger generally emerges from unresolved conflicts and if left unchanneled, nonproductive feelings ensue.

Let's analyze your bitterness for a moment. Did your doctor fail to listen or to spend the needed time with you to work out your problem? Did you feel that you were unimportant? Did you seek the help of several physicians who didn't seem to care? Are you living a life of chronic pain and still do not know why? Ultimately, did you give the system a fair chance or were you simply seeking "the cure?"

All of these questions are important and your honest answers can help resolve the frustrations that you have been harboring. Such feelings can help you pinpoint specific elements that can be partially responsible for fostering the ongoing nature of your suffering. In any event, the act of recognizing your frustrations is a very positive initial step if you allow yourself to channel your energies productively. Even if you cannot resolve all of your negative feelings regarding the medical profession, take the time to rethink your experiences. If they were positive, you wouldn't be reading this book. Something was obviously missing.

Use your energy to start fresh and develop a new foundation. It's impossible to be a good consumer if you can't identify or delineate the qualities of the product you wish to purchase. A logical beginning includes taking the time to conceptualize the very best product imaginable. A vague idea is not acceptable, as you obviously have a lot at stake. Remember, you must learn how to help yourself. As stated previously, the "cure me" approach must be forever erased from your memory bank. Your new perspective must be positive and productive.

Let's spend a few moments reviewing the types of practitioners available in the field of chronic pain management. Health care providers are extremely diverse and many are willing to see chronic pain sufferers. They adhere to different disciplines represented by schools of medicine, osteopathy, chiropractic and podiatry, to name just a few. In addition to family practitioners and internists, the field is represented by different areas of specialization, such as neurology, anesthesiology, orthopedics, neurosurgery, physiatry, rheumatology and psychiatry. Behavioral approaches are typically enlisted by psychologists, counselors, biofeedback therapists, hypnotherapists, social workers, drug and alcohol rehabilitation counselors, dieticians and the clergy. Physical rehabilitation is offered by physical and occupational therapists, personal fitness trainers, exercise physiologists and massage therapists. Substantial therapeutic overlap exists and the borders of service and specialization are progressively becoming more obscure. An increasing variety of options awaits you, as each discipline stakes its claim in the arena of pain management.

Before considering any of the above disciplines, let's refocus on your objective, which is clearly to become pain-free. Regardless of where you begin, two elements must be addressed. These are, as you would now expect, the mind and the body. Dealing with one without the other guarantees failure. It is not logical even to consider reprogramming just one of these elements while disregarding the other. Treating the entire person is the essence of success. Prior to exploring the holistic method, let's review some personal experiences utilizing the traditional approach.

Failure Of The Traditional Approach

After completing a neurology residency, I entered private practice with aspirations of helping my patients to enjoy the best health possible. My early experiences were diverse and many individuals with a host of disorders sought my attention. It became apparent early on that the most frustrating aspect of my practice was treating individuals with chronic pain disorders, such as headaches and back pain. Despite the use of the latest medicines suggested for each disorder and following medical text book recommendations explicitly, many patients continued to suffer. I was unable to help many of my patients. This account reflects the sad, realistic and frustrating experiences of many physicians who treat chronic pain patients. As I searched for a better approach, I reviewed my patients' experiences.

The challenges of dealing with people suffering from chronic pain are immense and the failures are often disconcerting, not only for the patient but also for the physician. Dedicated colleagues from many disciplines report similar feelings. Most physicians can easily recognize a life that has been shattered by pain and suffering, but finding a cure often seems impossible. Many doctors, out of the frustration of not being able to cure these sufferers, eventually veer away from patients with chronic pain and refer them to other practitioners. Some continue to treat their patients with drug after drug, realizing all too well that no medication will change such a person's life. At times, narcotics or addictive agents are prescribed to squelch the patients' complaints.

Some physicians become cynical and attribute their failures to the patient's lack of cooperation or their potential for monetary gain, which can be derived from workman's compensation benefits or insurance settlements. They refer to these individuals as "professional patients." It is unfortunate for honest individuals that such behavior does exist. However, I believe that the overwhelming majority of chronic pain patients are genuinely suffering on many levels.

Diagnosing a syndrome or recognizing the physical and psychological elements represents only a starting point. These issues must be addressed by incorporating a logical and structured treatment plan. The pain practitioner dedicated to this endeavor must accept the role of coach, not healer. Successful treatment is possible only if a doctor assumes this role. When physicians are ready and willing to work as a member of a team with a patient, meaningful alliances naturally develop and mature.

A logical approach, considering the diversity of elements in a chronic pain disorder, is to enlist the help of allied health professionals who can lead the patient in the proper direction. Such is the case for many practices, as patients are referred out for physical therapy and psychological services. The results, however, for chronic pain sufferers are often disappointing.

Victims of chronic pain are often initially resistant to an outside referral, especially for psychological counseling. The issue is uncomfortable. Just bringing up the subject of seeing a psychologist or counselor may potentially result in loss of trust. Sometimes the patient becomes upset and leaves the doctor's practice. As a result, the physician often does not wish to insinuate that the patient has a psychological problem. To worsen matters, many individuals dread returning home to tell their spouse or loved-one that they are scheduled to see a "shrink."

It is not surprising after an extensive workup that many people are disappointed to hear that no overt pathology is uncovered and that a psychological component may be present. It is a sad commentary that so many patients are treated for many disorders with pharmacotherapy alone, while the physician senses all along that a major source of stress is triggering or worsening an array of symptoms.

In defense of the doctor, physicians have not been traditionally taught to tackle these problems with a multidisciplinary approach. Unfortunately, practicing medicine with a narrow focus frequently results in excessive prescriptions of anxiolytics or "nerve pills," rather than addressing the underlying issues. Reviewing the financial statements of certain pharmaceutical companies supports the contention that such an approach is the rule, not the exception.

When an individual finally agrees to a referral, rarely does the counselor receive a copy of the patient's initial consultation or have the opportunity to discuss the patient with the referring physician. The reason for the visit is often provided by the pain sufferer and is almost always tempered by a host of preconceived notions or associations. The patient, who may have developed a long-standing rapport with his doctor, now perceives being thrust head on into the clutches of a new adversary who manipulates the mind and uncovers the darkest secrets. The experience is considered to be painful and embarrassing even before seeing the counselor. This association is difficult to reprogram and failure to return for a follow up visit may be inevitable.

An outside referral to a physical therapist can be extremely valuable under the proper circumstances. However, this approach sometimes leads to frustration. Chronic pain victims require specialized treatment programs, as well as a great deal of patience and interest. The physical therapist and rehabilitation setting must be geared to that individual. In today's world of technological advances, many physical therapists have dedicated themselves to specific areas of rehabilitation, such as sports injuries or strokes. The chronic pain victim may feel out of place in such a setting.

The most common mode of referral to a physical therapist is in the form of a prescription for therapy, without a comprehensive program being specified. Frequently, the therapist does not receive a call from the referring doctor or a detailed note documenting the history, findings, diagnosis, or overall treatment plan. In many cases, the therapist is expected to diagnose the problem and design a treatment strategy, which sometimes challenges the physician's diagnosis. Conflicts have a tendency to arise out of differences in opinion or terminology. Mixed signals promote lack of confidence. To complicate matters further, in many settings, the patient sees a different therapist with a unique perspective each time. All too often, the chronic pain patient returns to the physician for a monthly checkup, stating that physical therapy was discontinued two weeks ago, as the sessions were worsening the pain. The declaration is news to the physician, as the therapist's note is still en route.

The results of treating a victim of chronic pain in such a fashion are less than desirable. Treatment strategies carried out by any number of practitioners simultaneously can often be unsuccessful when communications are less than optimal. Generally, adequate time is not taken to appropriately discuss a patient's progress among the practitioners. The pain sufferer often receives impressions and directives that appear to be conflicting.

Each failed treatment attempt is not easily discarded from one's repertoire of experiences. Such failures have a tendency to add to the detrimental programming of the person. Such associations progressively become more deeply imbedded as history repeats itself and pessimism and frustration sets the stage for the likely failure of any future treatment endeavor.

Convergent Therapy

No one medical specialty has uncovered all of the clues for treating the chronic pain sufferer. Even the traditional independent medical practice, extended to include referrals to multiple disciplines, can be highly ineffective. In view of these failures, which largely stem from poor communication and ineffective organization of the therapeutic program, the concept of "convergent therapy" was introduced.

According to Webster, the word *convergent* signifies "the tendency to move toward one point or to approach each other, coming together." I presented this concept in a paper published a few years ago in the *Journal of Neurological and Orthopedic Medicine and Surgery. Convergent therapy* signifies the unification of various medical disciplines to produce an allied, coordinated effort for the purpose of treating a patient in the most effective manner possible. Individual

152

approaches are utilized concurrently to evoke a synergistic effect. The term *synergistic* suggests that the sum or total is equal to more than just the additive effects of the respective components. In other words, the benefits derived from a team far exceed the additive effects of individuals working alone.

Approaches for treating chronic pain patients vary considerably. Yet despite the diversity of perspectives, three components of an effective pain program are essential. These are represented by the medical, physical and psychological disciplines, which can be incorporated in a variety of ways, depending on the overall design of the program.

The Medical Approach

In our center, the medical approach is led by a physician, notably a neurologist or anesthesiologist/pain management specialist. The following is a procedural outline for my center. Our medical approach is based on accurate diagnosis, coupled with the organization and management of individualized treatment regimens.

The patient, prior to engaging in any treatment endeavor, begins our program with a thorough history and physical examination, performed by the physician/team leader who carefully reviews all available medical records. Although further tests are occasionally warranted, the majority of chronic pain sufferers have been worked up extensively by multiple practitioners in the past. It is not uncommon for the physician to spend at least an hour with the patient on the first visit. This, of course, depends upon the complexity of the issues presented. The team leader spends a great deal of time with the subject, carefully and thoroughly discussing the basis for the diagnosis as well as the details of the proposed treatment plan.

Medical issues covered include a careful survey of past and present medications, including over-the-counter drugs. The quantities consumed of each are carefully outlined. The physician openly addresses the addictive potential, as well as side effects and effectiveness of medicines presently used. A discussion of rebound effects takes place when applicable. The decision to stop or taper the use of a drug carries with it an obligation to present a logical rationale for doing so. If new medicines are to be prescribed, a straightforward explanation of benefits, side effects and drug interactions is presented. If injections are to be used in the form of intravenous, intramuscular, or spinal blocks, the physician considers and delves into the fears and misunderstandings that the patient may be harboring. We attempt to address these feelings with utmost patience and understanding.

Other medical issues deserve attention as well. If the patient is smoking, drinking alcohol, or ingesting illicit substances, a plan for reduction and eventual cessation is presented along with an explanation of the deleterious effects of each. In certain cases, medications are prescribed to counter withdrawal effects. Diet is also addressed and a discussion of the nutritional effects and specific food triggers ensues. At times, a specific diet is presented, depending on the patient's presentation. Dietary considerations are not overlooked in any patient.

The physician carefully reviews issues related to family, employment and, of course, stress. Therapeutic decisions take into consideration the opinions of other team members who are likely to learn more about the patient in specific areas. In addition to being provided with a reasonable prognosis, the patient does not leave the physician's office after the first visit without a comprehensive understanding of what to expect and what is expected. It is emphasized that the treating physician does not hand out "cures" and the patient should understand the necessity of taking an active, rather than a passive, role for recovery. Finally, the individual is given instructions regarding when and how to contact the physician for routine matters or emergencies.

The doctor leading a coordinated team must be familiar with all aspects of concurrent care. An open and frequent line of communication must exist in order to avoid potential pitfalls or setbacks. Details regarding the management of the "convergent" approach will be discussed later.

The Physical Approach

The physical aspect of therapy typically covers details such as movement, spasm, weakness, altered range of motion and diminished stamina. In our center, a licensed physical therapist heads a team dedicated to these components. A well-rounded program should include passive and active therapies, in addition to training and instruction in areas such as posture and movement. The physical approach, in our program, begins with a comprehensive evaluation by a physical therapist who discusses his findings with the patient and jointly develops a treatment strategy with the physician.

Typical passive modalities of therapy include heat or cold, ultrasound, various forms of electrical stimulation, massage and traction. Each has distinct advantages and disadvantages and are tolerated better by some than others. Most programs enlist the use of several modalities concurrently. In many cases, we provide training in the home use of certain passive procedures used in the center such as the application of hot packs or transcutaneous electrical stimulation (TENS) devices.

Active therapeutic modalities are based on personally tailored exercise programs. As discussed in Chapter 4, the chronic pain sufferer initially hesitates to begin an exercise program, believing that any form of movement may worsen pain. A deliberate, yet gentle and progressive approach is needed to reprogram this contention. Simple stretching to increase range of motion and to diminish muscle spasm may be enlisted at first. Later, progressive exercise and aerobic conditioning is possible in many cases. The effectiveness of a program is often based on the therapist's ability to inspire and encourage the patient to become more active.

Along with a responsive therapist, another important component of our physical approach is based on a structured program developed to teach the patient how to move. The concept may seem simple at first, yet the complexity of posture and motion is truly astounding. Incorrect or inefficient movements or postures can often serve as immense stumbling blocks. Understanding and recreating the postures of work or specific activities is essential and the patient should be directed toward increasing self-awareness. Wonderful programs have been developed to address these issues. In our Center, "Awareness Through Movement" is emphasized and taught by a certified Feldenkrais practitioner. The process of awareness, however, is emphasized through all aspects of our physical therapy program. Mind and body are not disassociated.

In order to achieve overall success, the entire team must have the flexibility and willingness to alter a treatment strategy immediately if necessary. Small adjustments within a program can turn potential failure into success. In addition, the patient should be followed by a specific therapist whenever possible, as maintaining a natural flow and continuity of care encourages progress.

The Psychological Approach

In the development of the "convergent" model, psychological processes must not be overlooked. Many programs utilize the services of counselors, psychologists or social workers to help the patient understand such issues and to develop strategies to become pain-free. It is important to note that most chronic pain programs are not based on traditional, lengthy psychoanalysis. Instead, a logical behavioral approach works more efficiently. Patients should interact with the counselor to uncover conflicts as well as sources of anger and frustration.

We use a practical approach to help the patient understand how certain issues, feelings or programmed responses may trigger pain. The patient is expected to play an active role in reprogramming pain through exercises and personal assignments designed to facilitate recovery. Our counselor also follows the subject's involvement in other areas of the program and covers issues such as diet, smoking and activity. The team focuses on inspiring the patient to persevere.

Disturbing issues from the past eventually surface and are dealt with in practical terms. The understanding or resolution of these traumatic experiences is not sufficient for the pain sufferer. The counselor must recognize the programmed responses that originally evolved from such experiences and continue to plague the sufferer. The baggage from the past must be converted into useful insights and the patient's physiological responses to a variety of stresses must be channeled effectively.

Hence, biofeedback is incorporated into the pain management program to provide a framework for self-control. Two objectives are generally specified. The first is the overall control of certain physiological responses which are injurious to the patient and which maintain the ongoing nature of the syndrome. The second is to provide a personal tool that can be willfully recruited to counter a painful attack. The subject is encouraged to understand these principles and to integrate biofeedback exercises into home or work settings. The value of such training must be discussed in the context of the subject's presentation.

Synergy In Pain Care

The elements of specialization must be organized and integrated into an overall pain treatment program. Synergy evolves naturally when communications are maintained throughout the disciplines. The key to the "convergent" approach is that the patient is not sent in different directions. Medical practitioners converge on the patient. The program is not spread across the boundaries of medical practices, nor hampered by conflicting explanations. The patient does not become a messenger between health care providers, as all medical records are readily available to the entire team. Treatment decisions are based on a collaborative approach, with each team member contributing essential insights, personal observations and impressions. The patient develops a level of comfort with the team that is reinforced by each discipline. Predictably, the overall effect is enhanced by the development of a sense of security within the patient.

The program's medical director acts as the head coach. He leads the team, moderates meetings and conferences and serves as the individual's advocate. This coach can only accomplish his mission with the cooperation and suggestions of the other coaches on the team. At times, when a specific obstacle is encountered, a team meeting with the patient and family promotes a multifaceted discussion that often breaks through even the toughest barriers.

Most patients are pleasantly surprised with such an approach. The comprehensive nature of this method requires, as one would expect, a firm commitment from the pain sufferer. Some people, however, are not ready for a such a challenge, which in reality is all-encompassing. Others find peace and solitude in this type of a cooperative effort, which has the potential to lead them to an improved quality of life. As a neurologist, the experience of utilizing the *convergent* technique has produced positive results beyond my expectations for the majority of chronic and refractory pain patients. The *convergent* environment enhances communications, heightens patient confidence, and promotes the reestablishment of normalcy for our patients.

You are probably wondering how to find a similar approach in your area. Many pain centers are based on the principles of *convergent* therapy. It is important to realize, however, that all pain centers and practitioners do not operate in this fashion. You should not rely purely on advertisements or telephone book listings, and you must be prepared to ask specific questions prior to engaging in any program. Most often, a nurse coordinator or practice manager can provide important information on the phone. At times, a well-prepared brochure may provide the answers. It's important to realize that the quality of your decision may be based, to a significant degree, on the questions you ask. Most important, however, is the fact that you are satisfied with the responses and wholeheartedly believe that the program is right for you. Consider asking some of the following questions prior to beginning any new program.

1. Is the program multidisciplinary?
2. What specialties are available and what are the backgrounds and credentials of the practitioners?
3. What types of non-drug therapies are utilized?
4. What modalities of physical therapy are available?
5. What types of psychological services are provided?
6. Is biofeedback included in the therapeutic regimen?
7. How is the program coordinated? How do the various disciplines interact?

An initial consultation with the physician/team leader should be performed prior to finalizing your decision. Consider asking yourself the following questions after seeing the doctor:

160

1. Did the practitioner spend the necessary time to carefully review my case and listen to my statements?
2. Was the examination thorough, covering the affected areas?
3. Was a diagnosis suggested and explained in terms I understand?
4. Do I understand my chances of recovery?
5. Did the doctor assume the role of coach, teacher or healer?
6. Did the physician's philosophy regarding the use of medication appear reasonable? Do I understand the potential side effects and benefits of the prescribed medicines? Are these acceptable to me?
7. Was the suggested manner of withdrawing or changing my present medicines explained in detail?
8. What were the doctor's opinions about physical and psychological therapies, as well as biofeedback? How are they integrated into the program?
9. How do I feel about the doctor's manner? Was it sincere and caring?
10. Am I comfortable with the availability of care on evenings and weekends? Is a team member available to answer my questions on a regular basis?
11. Do I feel comfortable dedicating myself to work closely with this physician/coach?

Take adequate time to review your answers. Consider discussing your feelings with a loved-one or close friend. Remember that your most important obligation is to yourself. Don't be afraid to trust your intuition. Be honest with yourself and try to set aside all of the negative feelings that have influenced you in the past. Is this physician the right one for you?

161

In his book, *How To Live Between Office Visits*, Dr. Bernie Siegel, focusing on the rapport between physician and patient, presents some interesting advice.

> I know some patients who have sat down and been totally sincere with the doctor, and this sincerity has led to tears and hugs on the part of both of them. If you initiate such sincerity and closeness and there is no response and you don't sense there is a human being on the other side of the desk, get up and get out.

Strive to be open-minded, intuitive and objective. Although you cannot be assured of arriving at the correct decision, you are now a more aware, informed and capable consumer. Commit yourself to this important decision and accept your active role in the process of learning to become pain-free. Although it's probably not yet apparent, you are already closer to your goal.

A Table With Three Legs

In order to better understand our approach, imagine a table supported by three legs. The first represents an accurate diagnosis coupled with comprehensive open-minded medical management. The second leg represents a combination of psychological approaches, including counseling and biofeedback. A structured program of passive and active physical therapy coupled with an emphasis on mind/body awareness serves as the third and final leg.

This holistic model promotes physical and mental well-being. Three legs are necessary to support our table. Removing just one would inevitably cause it to topple. In the very same manner, if any aspect of care is eliminated, the collective effort fails. Success is clearly attained in a synergistic fashion.

This comprehensive method of treating the entire person is practical and effective. A cooperative patient, coupled with a devoted, multidisciplinary team will produce results beyond your greatest expectations. If you accept this challenge with the goal of reestablishing normalcy in your life, pain can diminish and eventually disappear.

Convergent therapy represents the most logical method for treating the chronic pain sufferer. The overall effect is truly synergistic, as the value of the total approach certainly exceeds the additive effects of the respective components. An open-minded, creative, multidisciplinary strategy provides the greatest benefits in the field of chronic pain management.

Chapter 9

The Potential Within

Taking Action

Do not underestimate the power of the human spirit. No greater force exists to move mountains, conquer space or ensure world peace. It is not a deficiency in power that limits us, it is our lack of commitment and belief in ourselves.

By now, the principles presented in *Reprogramming Pain* have either resurrected a host of inner feelings to which you can relate or have turned you off to this approach. If the latter is the case, perhaps you believe that your pain is unique or entirely physical in nature. Your contentions may be based on resigning to a diagnosis such as a herniated disk or severe arthritis. In reality, your attitude may be further justified by the fact that you are already on disability, which erroneously acknowledges that you are destined to live with pain. Fortunately, however, you may be wrong!

You may be insistent that your pain cannot be controlled or even eliminated by the "convergent" method. Your understanding of a disorder that has become your greatest barrier to quality living may be far from the truth. Your inner beliefs can often be formidable obstacles in your path to recovery.

Do you realize that a vast number of individuals with arthritic or degenerative changes on x-rays do not suffer from associated pain? Are you aware of the fact that a phenomenal number of people who live without experiencing a day of back pain have bulging discs on their CT or MRI scans? Are you surprised by the fact that many victims of severe trauma, such as in motor vehicle accidents, are never limited by any remnant of pain? Is it news to you that many people with long histories of daily, incapacitating headaches, are now pain-free? Would you be surprised to learn that many of these individuals were initially in your boat--resistant to the concept that freedom from pain was well within their grasp?

I can assure you that all of these statements are true. The inspiration for writing this book was born out of feelings I personally experienced observing the remarkable improvements in the lives of many long-term pain sufferers who didn't originally believe they had the slightest chance of recovery. Even my initial doubts were dispelled by these incredible improvements.

The Power of the Human Spirit

Do not underestimate the power of the human spirit. No greater force exists to move mountains, conquer space, or ensure personal success. It is not a deficiency in power that limits us, it is our lack of commitment and belief in ourselves. The principal obstacles to your recovery lie within you, as programmed associations, hampering your will and spirit. We must learn to reprogram our approach to life in general! As James Allen once said in *As a Man Thinketh:*

> Man is made or unmade by himself;
> in the armory of thought he forges the
> weapons by which he destroys him-
> self; he also fashions the tools with
> which he builds for himself heavenly
> mansions of joy and strength and peace.
> By the right choice and true applica-
> tion of thought man ascends to the
> divine perfection.

It is difficult for many of us to abandon our reliance on medication and technology and look into ourselves for the answers. I am not asking you to disregard all of the technical advances in modern medicine. Rather, I hope you will understand that there are other important dimensions to be considered.

Getting started seems to require great effort. It's always simpler to retreat to our old habits, regardless of the consequences. It is often unsettling to begin any self-help endeavor and uncomfortable attempting to reprogram well-established beliefs and behaviors that are detrimental to our survival. Change is typically accepted with great difficulty as we are creatures of habit--good and bad, right and wrong.

167

It takes substantial commitment to overcome the inertia, or resistance, to any change. However, once in motion, strength appears to build progressively as obstacles are successively hurdled.

It should be obvious by now that I am committed to getting you started. I truly believe that once you have accepted this challenge and begin the process of learning to live a pain-free existence, your chances for success are excellent. I realize that you would not be reading this book had you not already overcome many seemingly overwhelming obstacles. Human nature, coupled with a dose of perseverance, provides the flexibility and fortitude to meet the countless challenges that you have already conquered. You will succeed in reestablishing normalcy in your life and thus defeat pain if you believe in yourself, think positively and pursue the right course. Thomas Hanna once said:

> Expectation is what carries us from the present into the future. As such, it is like the prow of a vessel nosing its way forward. The direction in which the prow is pointed determines the direction the vessel will go. The prow leads the movement of the vessel. If the prow points up, the vessel will follow in the same direction: upward. If the prow points down, the vessel will go downward. The course of our life follows our expectations in the same way that a vessel follows the direction of its prow.

Positive directives can often be undermined by negative feelings. There are so many reasons you've devised for not taking care of yourself. You might be too busy or involved in other problems. You may believe that you are unimportant and not worth the effort. You might justify your procrastination by convincing yourself that there is no help. You may have settled for a lifestyle that you're used to and somewhat comfortable with, even though it's painful.

You may be correct in one regard; an excuse always surfaces in a time of need. You must realize, as Donald Robert Perry Marquis once said, "Procrastination is the art of keeping up with yesterday." To forge ahead you must face the future, as yesterday is no more than a memory that can impede your progress.

Sometimes we program ourselves to live within the confines of our excuses, believing that our problems are truly insurmountable. In fact, you've probably developed steadfast responses for why you're not exercising, watching your diet or even trying another approach for pain. As a result, you may have arrived at the conclusion that there is no hope. After all, you've failed in the past and those horrible disappointments probably felt even worse than your present situation. When all of the cards are finally on the table, fear of failure is probably the true reason for not getting started. Of all the emotions we experience, fear is certainly our most destructive programming tool, capable of inducing a terminal state known as *quitting*.

We have the tendency to shy away from potentially painful experiences, even when there is an opportunity to improve the quality of our lives. Fragile and easily misled, we eventually settle into believing that we're better off where we are. The risks of failure somehow tend to outweigh the prospects of success. You may be existing without a positive dream in sight.

For the chronic pain sufferer, despair and fear of failure is the rule, not the exception. However, no time is better than now to break that rule. Begin by believing in yourself. The power to heal yourself lies within you. The problem, however, is that you have never given yourself an adequate chance. You have the capacity for change, if you put your mind to it. You must begin by breaking the shackles of procrastination! The programmed associations of the past that control you must be reprogrammed.

By now, you are probably aware of unhealthy past associations and have a reasonable idea of where your problem areas lie. Remember, you are not alone; help certainly exists. As an enlightened consumer, you are now in a better position to tackle your problems and change the course of your life. You must play an active role in your recovery. Relish the fact that you can now enjoy the most wonderful opportunity of your life--to seek the very best help possible.

Your progress will certainly spill over to those around you; your loved ones and your friends. Your gains in many ways will be theirs. A wonderful relationship with another person can be the key to restoring your faith in mankind and yourself. My wife, Karen, has taught me about life through her never-questioning faith in God. Always seeing the positive and often blinded to the negative, she finds happiness in even the simplest aspects of life and sets an example of respect and compassion for all creatures. Re-exploring your relationship with a loved-one or extending yourself to others, even in a time of personal need, can facilitate the rebirth of your own faith in yourself. I often recommend volunteering to help others, even when you are hurting, as a means of reestablishing a sense of pride, self-esteem and faith.

When I explain the *convergent* approach, some individuals are immediately turned off as the concept at first appears too simple. After all, there are no gimmicks. The beauty of this strategy for reprogramming yourself is the innate simplicity of the method. The greatest philosophers of the world have acknowledged that the most wonderful concepts of life are, in fact, simple.

Many patients, after having successfully reprogrammed their pain, tearfully admit to me that they did not initially believe that such an elementary approach could succeed when years of medication, and even multiple surgeries, led to one failure after another.

Another excuse for not taking this important step is based on the realization that such a program requires too much commitment. "Convergent therapy" and the process of reprogramming pain is certainly not the "quick fix" for your problem. Some people are frankly disappointed when the "miracle drug" is not prescribed. In fact, for some, just the consideration of reducing medication consumption, or for that matter, alcohol or tobacco use, remains a price too great to pay for health. These individuals do not realize that they have the capacity to change and to reestablish a sense of balance in their lives.

Priorities among individuals vary considerably and each one of us has to balance the scales and accept the consequences of our decisions. I adhere to the time-proven observation that we achieve nothing in life of lasting value instantly. The greatest satisfaction in life is not realized by achieving a goal, it is the process of getting there that provides the most important lessons and rewards.

As positive as I am that this approach represents the best path to a pain-free state, I am frequently astounded with our results. Individuals have come to our center with histories of suffering that have been so prolonged and so unimaginable that even I doubt that the slightest chance of restoring quality of life exists. When the team does in fact finally break through to such patients, the most wonderful metamorphosis develops in front of our eyes. These individuals truly provide our greatest rewards and reaffirm our belief in the power of the human spirit.

When I review such a patient's progress, I am frequently unable to pinpoint the precise nature of that which prompted the phenomenal transformation. Each person is clearly unique and no two individuals respond in the same way to any aspect of a holistic program. After studying this issue deliberately in several patients, I have arrived at the following conclusion: Reestablishing normalcy in a person's life and thus eliminating pain predictably results from identifying and utilizing the patient's own strengths as the primary force leading to recovery. Perhaps the best healers are trusted coaches who effectively reprogram people to help themselves. As stated in *The Prophet*, by Kahlil Gibran:

> Your pain is the breaking of the shell
> that encloses your understanding. Even

as the stone of the fruit must break, that its heart may stand in the sun, so must you know pain. And could you keep your heart in wonder at the daily miracles of your life, your pain would not seem less wondrous than your joy. And you would accept the seasons of your heart, even as you have always accepted the seasons that pass over your fields. And you would watch with serenity through the winters of your grief. Much of your pain is self-chosen. It is the bitter potion by which the physician within you heals your sick self. Therefore trust the physician, and drink his remedy in silence and tranquility: For his hand, though heavy and hard, is guided by the tender hand of the Unseen, and the cup he brings, though it burn your lips, has been fashioned of the clay which the Potter has moistened with His own sacred tears.

Bringing out the best in people often works wonders. The resultant ripples in the pond of life are manifested on many levels and the patient is not the only one who benefits. Physicians are often inspired by their patients. In an attempt however, to practice effective medicine, physicians sometimes lose sight of the most important issues.

The Pitfalls of Scientific Conclusions

Many well-trained scientists and physicians began with the belief that if a finding could not be proven through a "double-blinded" study, it was immediately invalidated. A double blinded study is one in which neither the experimenters nor the subjects know who is receiving the real treatment. A substance with no presumed effect is used as a basis for comparison with a new drug. This substance is typically referred to as a *placebo*. For many, this term is probably synonomous with a sugar pill. When researchers test the effects of a pain medication in a group of people, a placebo is given to what we term the *control* group. The published conclusions for a new drug are based on statistical differences comparing results in the *experimental* group (subjects taking the *real* drug) to the *control* group.

Such logic appears straightforward, yet the results are not. Despite the fact that typically 20-70% of subjects who receive placebos in double-blinded studies improve, we look no further. To complicate matters, a significant percentage of subjects given placebos predictably develop side-effects! Medical scientists seem to disregard the importance of the fact that so many people improve or worsen even when they are not given the *real* drug. We seem to explain away such conclusions by assuming that placebo responders are not truly suffering in the first place and that their manifestations of illness are no more than *psychosomatic* complaints. Such conclusions are based upon ignorance of the true mind/body link.

As you have seen in prior chapters, one's belief system is inseparable from one's physical responses. When you worry, detrimental signals are immediately sent to end organs through a complex system of peptides described in Chapter 2. You have also seen through Dr. Lee Berk's outstanding work that laughter objectively translates into improved immune performance. It is frightening that many physicians and scientists have failed to realize that the ultimate value of a drug or treatment may be primarily based on the subject's belief system, or the manner in which the therapy is delivered. It is not surprising that certain therapeutic endeavors work extremely well in the hands of one group and seem to fail miserably when used by others.

In effect, when an individual experiencing pain *believes* that he or she is being given a promising drug or treatment, a very real biochemical and physiological change results. Considering the fact that 20-70% of subjects receiving placebos improve, imagine how much better we would feel if we didn't have to contend with the adverse side effects of real drugs. Since one's state of "mind" is clearly a significant determinant of pain control and health, we should be focusing our attention on improving the physician-patient bond and promoting positive expectations for our patients.

An important issue to resolve at this point is the basis for and the location of that which we refer to as the *mind*. Candace Pert, Ph.D., former Chief of the Section on Brain Biochemistry of the Clinical Neuroscience Branch at the National Institute of Mental Health and the discoverer of the opiate receptor describes the mind/body link in practical terms. She refers to neuropeptides and their receptors as "the biochemical correlates of emotion." When Bill Moyers in *Healing and The Mind* asked her to describe the mind, she responded:

175

> The mind is some kind of enlivening
> energy in the information realm throughout
> the brain and body that enables the
> cells to talk to each other, and the outside
> to talk to the whole organism.

Understanding the essence of health at the cellular level may be the ultimate key to a quality existence. Dr. Pert approaches *health* in the following manner:

> The word "health" itself is so inter-
> esting because it comes from a root
> that means "whole." Part of being a
> healthy person is being well-integrated
> and at peace, with all of the systems
> acting together.

A View From Within

The establishment of a well-integrated, peaceful and balanced state promotes a pain-free and meaningful existence. Allow me to take a few moments to share a wonderful experience with you. A few years ago I enjoyed the opportunity of caring for a young person whose life had been severely affected by debilitating headaches, neck pain and dizziness. Her course in our program was basically uneventful, as she progressively learned to eliminate her pain. She worked diligently and never complained about or even questioned any of the team's suggestions. In fact, she was so cooperative that no stumbling stone was ever brought to my attention throughout her treatment. On her last day in our program, with tears in her eyes, she thanked me for having guided her through the process of overcoming the suffering which had once destroyed the quality of her life. She placed a paperback in my hand, as a simple token of her appreciation. I promised her that I would find time to read the book, not realizing, however, the true value of this gift.

Three days passed, as a wealth of knowledge lay concealed within the covers of a small blue paperback on my night table. Once I started reading, the story about a seemingly simple "Rag Picker" revealed more to me about life, the power of the human spirit and the act of inspiring others to help themselves than anything I had ever read. This book, *The Greatest Miracle In The World* by Og Mandino, is truly one of the most valuable works, or perhaps gifts, of the modern era.

Through a flowing, mystical storyline, Mandino reveals the strengths and potential of each human being. A wonderful and simple method is presented to literally REPROGRAM the human spirit to soar to heights limited only by one's imagination.

Og Mandino's encouragement is set forth with a wonderfully smooth, simple and self-reflective style. He states:

> Be patient with your progress. To count
> your blessings with gratitude, to pro-
> claim your rarity with pride, to go an
> extra mile and then another, these acts
> are not accomplished in the blinking
> of an eye. Yet, that which you ac-
> quire with most difficulty you retain

the longest; as those who have earned a fortune are more careful of it than those by whom it was inherited. And fear not as you enter your new life. Every noble acquisition is attended with its risks.

After reading this book, I personally handed every member of our clinical staff a copy to read and study. Since that time, we have recommended *The Greatest Miracle In The World* to many of our patients as one of the best steps for beginning a journey toward a pain-free existence. I prescribe this book to all of you, as one of the greatest motivational tools you will ever have the pleasure to utilize.

I am truly indebted to Mr. Mandino and my patient for one of the most important inspirations of my life. His faith serves as a powerful engine for his works. In reflecting on the Almighty's perspective, Mandino states:

Be proud. You are not the momentary whim of a careless creator experimenting in the laboratory of life. You are not a slave of forces that you cannot comprehend. You are a free manifestation of no force but mine, of no love but mine. You were made with a purpose.

A Higher Force

I suppose there are times when each one of us cannot seem to develop the strength or purpose necessary to get started. It's impossible to judge any person's effort, as so many mental roadblocks exist within us. Our preprogrammed responses, based on years of negative experiences and hardships, are difficult to overcome. Most often, we are not aware of the forces that prevent us from helping ourselves. There are times when we truly do need help and we must look to a higher force. I acknowledge the fact that I need that force to practice medicine. For that matter, I believe that it is impossible to attain anything of value in life without faith.

Many people do not realize that failure to believe in one's self is incompatible with faith in God. For them, the human spirit surprisingly appears to occupy a different realm. Perhaps they do not realize that the essence of the Almighty is within us and losing faith in yourself is contradictory to believing in a higher force. It's tragic to realize that so many victims of chronic pain have given up on themselves and have lost their once-cherished bond with God.

As a scientist, I have arrived at the realization that many of my observations over the years are not easily explained in purely physical terms. Countless cases have been documented describing spontaneous remissions and cures that have been described by many as miracles. I am convinced that there is a force that binds all of us; that somehow we are all in the soup of life together. The focus of this section is not on religion, What I am about to share links spirituality and the mind to the practice of medicine.

A wonderful technique for developing a closer link with the truth that abounds within and connects the entire universe through the Almighty is meditation. Although documented throughout the ages, meditation is just now becoming an accepted tool for reestablishing health. Deepak Chopra, M.D., a prominent and respected pioneer in this field, describes this art eloquently in his book *Ageless Body Timeless Mind*:

> You can learn to take your awareness into the region of timelessness at will - meditation is the classic technique for mastering this experience. In meditation the active mind is withdrawn to its source; just as this changing universe had to have a source beyond change, your mind, with all its restless activity, arises from a state of awareness beyond thought, sensation, emotion, desire, and memory. ...You sense that the infinite is everywhere.

Perhaps the most straightforward guide to meditation is found in writings of Herbert Benson, M.D., of Harvard University's Mind/Body Medical Institute. In his bestselling book, *The Relaxation Response*, Dr. Benson clearly outlines the keys to using meditation for improving one's health. He presents four basic and essential elements: a quiet environment, an object to dwell upon, a passive attitude and a comfortable position. In a subsequent work, *Beyond The Relaxation Response*, he clearly binds the elements of spirituality to the act of redefining personal health.

Dr. Benson is an outstanding and dedicated scientist who introduced the true essence of meditative techniques to mainstream medicine. With deep feeling, compassion and utmost respect for all people, he has emphasized the value of incorporating one's own spirituality into personal wellness. His books demonstrate not only phenomenal insights into mind/body healing but also represent a selfless gift that has the potential to transform your life beyond your greatest expectations.

You may be saying to yourself that there is no proof that such practices ever really produce results. You are not alone, as your skepticism is shared by others. Yet over the last few years, we have learned that meditation has its place in the practice of medicine. Dean Ornish, M.D., president and director of the Preventive Medicine Research Institute at the School of Medicine, University of California, San Francisco, has successfully developed a program to reverse coronary artery blockages. His remarkable accomplishments were based on a program consisting of exercise, diet and meditation. In *Healing and The Mind*, Dr. Ornish describes his impressions:

> I began this work with a certain degree of skepticism. But what I am coming away with is an appreciation for how powerful the mind is in affecting our health, for better or for worse. As physicians, we can, deliberately or inadvertently, increase the negative effects of the mind on the body - but we can

also use the mind to have a healing
effect on the heart.

Dr. Ornish's model for patients with coronary artery disease
has received worldwide attention and is changing the minds
of many skeptics. If such an approach can improve blood
flow to the heart, imagine what it can do for your pain.

Based on the belief that we are all connected cosmi-
cally, we must assume responsibility for our own actions
and their effects on others. The contention that the doctor's
belief system is as important as the patient's has been promoted by many pioneers in this field such as Norman Cousins, Bernie Siegel, Lee Pulos, Wayne Dyer and Larry Dossey.
The physician's belief system and its role in the healing process
is examined in *Healing Words* by Larry Dossey, M.D. His
conclusions are summed up as follows:

> The power of the physician's belief
> system to shape the patient's responses
> to therapy is akin to prayer. Both prayer
> and belief are nonlocal manifestations
> of consciousness, because both can
> operate at a distance, sometimes out-
> side the patient's awareness. Both affirm
> that "it's not all physical," and both
> can be used adjunctively with other
> forms of therapy.

Healing Words presents an extensive compilation of controlled
clinical trials, studying the effects of prayer on healing. Dr.

Dossey's book is an eye-opening experience. As a physician, I never believed that the day would come when spirituality, meditation, guided imagery, prayer and soul-searching would be considered valuable methodologies by prominent members of medical profession. I am certain that most of my colleagues do not welcome this perspective or are hesitant to say so. My life has been greatly enriched by such wonderful and universal insights and my hopes and aspirations for those I treat have been elevated to a higher level.

Success is Yours

Your willingness to persevere is the essence of success and the nature of your approach will predictably determine your accomplishment. You must always look within yourself for the strength to continue, for your initiative can only be fueled by your passion. Don't hold back in your quest for a new life. As Og Mandino effectively stated:

> The mediocre never goes another mile, for why should he cheat himself, he thinks. But you are not mediocre. To go another mile is a privilege you must appropriate by your own initiative. You cannot, you must not avoid it. Neglect it, do only as little as the others, and the responsibility for your failure is yours alone.

You must believe in yourself and assume the responsibility of following through in order to reach your goal of a pain-free state. So much can be learned along the way if your attitude is positive and you have faith in yourself. Do not remain stagnant! Take a stand, believe in yourself and start anew. Lee Pulos, Ph.D., and Gary Richman summed it up beautifully in *Miracles and Other Realities*: "Belief in nothing is the most confining belief of all."

Chapter 10

Reprogramming Pain

10 Logical Steps

Ultimately, you alone have the power to shape your destiny. Your decision to live without chronic pain must represent the conscious effort of your entire being.

The prospect of attaining a pain-free existence may seem like an impossible dream at first. Given the complexity of the issues to be tackled, even the act of getting started may seem frightfully overwhelming. This is often the case for any goal of similar magnitude or value.

Projects of immense complexity can only be completed through the development of a precise and logical strategy. Such accomplishments are only possible by carefully dividing the entire undertaking into individual components and designating specific tasks in a logical manner. The key to your ultimate success is based on properly identifying each step, carrying out a reasonable plan and maintaining the will to persevere.

Your level of understanding has gradually evolved to the critical point of placing your thoughts into motion. You have the power within you to rid yourself of pain if you set your mind to it. All of your well-conceived notions and revelations about your present state will vanish into oblivion, if you do not take action now!

Ten important steps will be presented in this chapter to provide the precise framework for developing a pain-free state. While there is room for creative design within this program, you must not consider skipping even one step. Remember to learn from your new experiences, as the journey itself may be more important than the final destination.

Step #1
Take Action!

A few years ago, a cherished friend and spiritual leader, Reverend Charles Henderson, presented me with a simple book entitled *Jacob The Baker, Gentle Wisdom For A Complicated World*, by Noah benShea. The universal wisdom of this book is delivered through a series of short questions and wonderful answers. My favorite chapter is only a few pages long and carries within it the most reasonable explanation for understanding why people have difficulty getting started. *"Building Fear"* is a story about a community leader who is worried about the meaning of a repetitive dream, in which he sees himself, after a long journey, facing the gates of a great city. A guard advises him that entrance is contingent upon properly answering two questions. The first question the soldier asks is:

> "What supports the walls of a city?"

> "That is easy," said Jacob. "Fear supports the walls of a city."

> "But what supports the fear?" asked the man. "For that is the second question."

> "The walls," answered Jacob. "The fears we cannot climb become our walls."

Jacob, through a deceptively simple dialogue, proposes that our personal limitations are often instilled by fear. Whether it be fear of the unknown or even fear of failure, we are easily stopped dead in our tracks. The boundaries or walls, which are subsequently self-imposed and personally limiting, maintain and even nurture fear. No better example exists than the fear of change that can serve as your most powerful jailor.

The fear of getting started is a programmed response that you must change. You have so much to gain by climbing over or even leveling the walls of your present existence and taking action for your personal well-being. If deep down within, you are not truly committed to the task at hand, consider rereading Chapter 9. Working through the remaining nine logical steps can bring the light at the end of the tunnel into full view.

Step #2
Perform a "Personal Reflections" Inventory

The process of defining a strategy for a pain-free existence can be most effectively shaped by assessing your present state. Discovering critical information about yourself and your condition can provide meaningful data for this endeavor. In order to set sail on a distant journey, you must first establish your present location as the primary position of reference. In the same manner, you must become keenly aware of your present condition, prior to effectively navigating the course to success.

You may have already completed a "Personal Reflections" inventory as you read Chapter 6. If not, please take the next few days to carefully review the questions and perspectives presented in that chapter for the purpose of developing a realistic personal assessment. If you did complete this step when you read the chapter, spend some important "quiet" time reviewing your answers. Don't frown on the fact that your initial ideas may have changed as you learned more about yourself. You are in the process of truly evolving as a more complete person and revising your assessment is a wonderful reflection of your continued self-awareness. Remember, no one is keeping score or grading your responses, as this is your personal viewing glass. In any event, I congratulate you for getting this far. You may, however, present your "Personal Reflections" inventory to a friend, loved-one or even a spiritual leader whom you respect. This can, at times, further refine and bring to the surface important details.

By now, you know whether or not you've crossed the line into the realm of chronic unremitting and refractory pain. Your "Personal Reflections" inventory tells the story. This profile will forever document your initial point of reference. Having completed this task, your accomplishments are substantial. Let's review them for a moment.

You carefully detailed your frustrations and losses in life and understand their overall impact on your being. You realize more clearly the specific effects of chronic pain on your life. You characterized your patterns of medication use and uncovered habits that are clearly detrimental to your health, serving as barriers to improvement. You revealed your innermost thoughts and frustrations regarding medical care received in the past and developed new insights for future considerations. You faced the issue of deciphering the basis for suffering in realistic terms. You looked in the mirror and saw yourself with new clarity and heightened focus. Most importantly, you faced your problems and know where you stand. You are now on the path to controlling your pain, rather than allowing it to control you.

Commend yourself for completing your "Personal Reflections" inventory, for you've taken the most difficult and courageous step in the process of freeing yourself from chronic pain. Facing the issues and seeing yourself for the very first time from a new and distinct vantage point requires great strength. Do not discard or cast away your personal inventory, as it will always be a diary of your progress. Take time to reread your statements regularly during your quest. Continue to add to your observations and always remember where you once were. Someday, you will look back and reread this soul-searching account of an individual whom you will fortunately no longer recognize as yourself.

Step #3
Study Your
Pain and Movement Patterns

Improved body awareness is the goal of Step 3. As discussed in Chapter 4, we have much to learn by developing an understanding of ourselves through our patterns of movement. "Personal Reflections" is a behavioral survey that has the potential to document your feelings and frustrations as well as your overall "emotional" status. In a similar manner, Step 3 will survey your "motional" status.

Prior to entering the realm of patterned movements, let's focus for now on your syndrome from a variety of perspectives. The factors to be studied include pain, spasm, numbness and limitation of range of motion. The most practical approach for this survey is to map your body, based on the way you feel, using the diagrams that follow. Please make some copies of these illustrations or trace them prior to proceeding.

Body Map

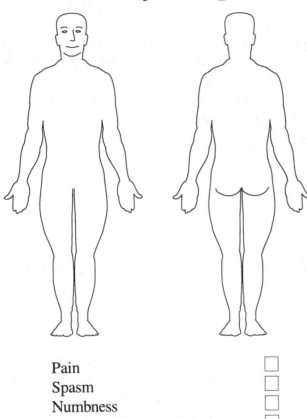

Pain ☐
Spasm ☐
Numbness ☐
Restricted Range of Motion ☐

For this important exercise, you will need four different colored pencils, crayons or markers. The colors must be distinct from each other and easily recognizable. Don't choose four shades of green, as each might not be clearly discernible. Find a quiet place and allocate approximately 15 minutes to perform this task.

Begin by coloring in the legend beneath the diagram which indicates the specific attribute assigned to each color. As an example, red could signify pain, blue for spasm, green for numbness and yellow for restricted range of motion. Start with pain and carefully color in the areas on the front and back views to signify what you feel. Take time and focus on each body part, prior to marking your map. Do not perform this activity from memory, as we are not interested in preconceived notions. This diagram must reflect exactly what you feel now! Review your work and fine tune it, if necessary. You may discard your map at any time and start again. Don't even consider asking for help from someone else; this assignment is yours alone. When you finish with pain, proceed to mark your diagram in a similar manner for spasm, numbness and limited range of motion.

For spasm, mark all the areas that feel tight and for numbness include attributes such as diminished feeling, tingling, pins and needles and even creeping-crawly sensations. Again, disregard how you felt in the past and focus only on the present. You might be saying to yourself that your body changes considerably as the day progresses. If this is the case, redraw your map at different intervals to reflect those variations. You may wish to have one for morning, noon and evening. In any event, never speculate about how you are going to feel, instead practice reading your body at this very moment.

Spend the next week reviewing your map each day and indicating changes when necessary. Feel free to add notes to your diagram at any time, as your reviews are critical to the process of understanding your body.

Once you have focused on precisely how you feel, create a list of activities similar to the one below. Feel free to ad lib wherever necessary. Your list should include your personal daily actions, which may include, yet not be limited to:

sitting	*lying on the couch*
bathing	*lying in bed*
shopping	*driving*
working	*standing*
walking	*bending*
lifting	*climbing stairs*

For each activity, note how your pain is affected, simply by indicating "better," "worse" or "no change." Perform this exercise at least three times in one week. After your tally is complete, cross off any action that is indicated by "better" or "no change." This will leave a list of only the activities that worsen your pain.

You have effectively mapped your body and developed greater self-awareness. You have also learned which specific movements or activities worsen your suffering. In reality, you have accomplished quite a bit, but let's not stop here. Beginning now, focus on one painful activity each day and gently experiment by changing the way you are doing it. Use a full-length mirror whenever possible to follow your actions. You may be amazed to find yourself walking tilted to one side or dragging one leg rather than lifting it, causing increased stress to other muscles or joints. In any event, try to gently change your position, speed or flow of movement. Experiment with some relaxing music while you're alone and calm. Most importantly, take your time and work with one activity at a time. This is not intended to be an exercise program, but rather a platform for heightened self-awareness.

Do not despair if you're not entirely successful, as your increased awareness will be extremely helpful when you present your personal findings to your physician or physical therapist. At times you might lead yourself to believe that a significant improvement is not occurring, as your perception of change is quite easily deceived. When in doubt, recheck your original body map and you may be delightfully surprised with your progress.

Step #4
Survey Your External Influences

This step is rather straightforward, yet requires some organized thought. As you recall from the early chapters of this book, our scope of outside influences extends to loved-ones, family, friends, business associates, health care providers and even the media. Our internal concept of pain and suffering is, to a significant extent, experiential, in that past experiences often condition or mold our present behaviors. The goal of Step 4 is to clearly separate your suffering and turmoil from the pain. By carefully dissecting your meaning of pain, you can learn to deal with it effectively using logical vantage points.

Feelings that appear to be simple, are often complex and not easily deciphered. For some, pain signifies loss of self-esteem, more than actual hurting. For others, it is the wrenching pit in your gut that seems to accompany any thought of failure. For all of us, pain carries a different connotation, which is truly multifaceted. Let's spend some valuable time trying to understand what pain really means to us.

In Chapter 3, we presented the "Reprogramming Pain Inventory," (RPI) to develop a vocabulary categorizing pain. You may wish to reread this section and perform your RPI prior to embarking on this important exercise. You should begin by setting aside some uninterrupted time to calmly reflect on your innermost feelings. New insights and revelations are bound to develop.

Close your eyes for a moment and breathe deeply, allowing your mind to wander for a few minutes before proceeding. Now, focus on the word *pain*. List each word that comes to mind on a sheet of paper. When you're finished, close your eyes again and let your mind float for a few moments. Then review your list and expand on it, adding new feelings and thoughts as you progress. You're accomplishing more than you can imagine.

Do not review your list again for at least a day. Use your time to work on the other steps for now. Tomorrow, take out your list and survey your key words. You may add to it any time. The goal of our exercise today is to focus on each term. Now for the tricky part! Allow your mind to wander and to freely associate. For each word, expand on it with the issue, conflict, person or activity to which it pertains. As an example, if you listed the word "anger," note to whom or what your anger is directed. What produced the "anger?" Was it your family, employer, doctor or your own action in the past? If the word is "shame," how did that feeling originate? Were you programmed to believe that pain was something to be ashamed of? Now is the time to sort out your past, even if it temporarily adds to your pain.

Dissecting a feeling into its respective components can provide you with the ability to achieve a goal previously thought to be impossible. Consider the following example that I recall from a story told to me as a child. It begins in days of old, when a father faces the decision of whom will be in charge of his estate when he dies. Wishing to give all three of his sons a fair chance, he devises a task to test their abilities. The object is simple; each son is given a bundle of sticks tied by some twine and is asked to break it in half. The first son, a mighty warrior, confidently grasps the sticks in his hands and bends as hard as possible. Despite his best efforts, the sticks remain intact. The second son, a world class athlete, props the bundle of sticks between two boulders and proceeds to jump on them with all his might, unfortunately to no avail. The third son, a mere writer of poetry, approaches the problem, contemplates the solution for a few moments and proceeds to untie the twine carefully, after which he easily breaks each stick, one at a time. Take this time to separate your feelings and to deal with them individually. As you can see, the key to success is clearly based on the approach.

Step #5
Face Ongoing Conflicts

We have the tendency to carry on our shoulders the excessive burdens of past experiences. This baggage contains unresolved conflicts that are true barriers to personal progress. The mere existence of such issues stunts our development. In fact, just the recollection of an unresolved issue conditions a troublesome response.

You really cannot take a meaningful step forward if you're locked in by past experiences. The purpose of this step is to finally come to terms with issues that are impeding your progress. You may have already developed insights regarding this matter in Step 4. Let's begin to focus on and resolve these potentially critical issues, conflicts or associations.

You must identify and come to reasonable terms with the conflicts in your life. We all have them, yet most often, we're not inclined to face these uncomfortable issues. Perhaps you're harboring sentiments related to a conversation or argument with your employer. Were you hurt by something that was said and is still reverberating in your mind? Were you once told that you would never succeed by someone you respected? Have you been led to believe that you will be living with pain indefinitely? Is there a situation in your life that continues to eat away at you?

It is not uncommon with this form of soul-searching to uncover conflicts with family members or loved-ones as a source of suffering. At times certain issues, which have marred your life, cannot be easily resolved. Unfortunately, rather than facing these painful relationships, we tend to distance ourselves from these issues. As a result, the conflict builds and worsens, rather than being resolved.

Your goal in Step 5 is to select three important conflicts in your life and resolve them. This may appear elementary at first, yet the successful completion of this endeavor may be more consuming than you can imagine. Within the three choices, you should address a relationship with a person. Your strategies might include the face-to-face resolution of an issue with someone who has hurt you. Discussing the problem with a member of the clergy or a counselor can often provide a helpful start. It may be reasonable, under certain circumstances, to approach the issue alone. However, if you're truly honest with yourself, you will probably realize your limitations and seek help when necessary.

You must document, in written form, the three conflicts of your choice and how you resolved or attempted to resolve them. You will be amazed with the overall difference in the way you feel when these burdens are finally lifted, as your efforts will be rewarded on many levels. Do not despair if success is not immediately apparent. If, after trying your best, the solution is not at hand, consider focusing on these issues when you seek help through the "convergent" model. Be assured that you will evolve into a more complete person when those issues that have eroded the surface of your being can no longer tear you apart. Anger does not wear well on you; learn to forgive!

Step #6
Incorporate Personal Strengths Into A Positive Attitude

It's only human nature to focus on our weaknesses, rather than on our strengths. The depression associated with chronic pain tarnishes almost any positive personal reflection. Step 6 is devised to polish your self-image with the luster of your past successes by uncovering your positive strengths and incorporating them into a new strategy.

As a pain practitioner, I can identify no better indicator of one's potential to attain a pain-free existence than a prior track record of success in almost any endeavor. I believe you can learn to resurrect dormant personal strengths and place them into action to attain almost any goal. Why not try harnessing that energy and developing the zeal to succeed?

In order to become pain-free, you must identify and activate the personal strengths that have worked for you in the past, while developing a positive and hopeful perspective. As James Allen stated in *As A Man Thinketh*, "Thoughts of courage, self-reliance and decision crystallize into manly habits, which solidify into circumstances of success, plenty, and freedom." Do not be afraid to rely on your own strengths and intuition. Study your accomplishments and learn from them, while allowing your past successes to give birth to new ones. Allow your strengths to work for you.

If at one time you were a great organizer, develop an organized approach for improving your life. If you were a good leader, enlist that sense of confidence you once experienced to lead yourself to success. If you were a good follower, find an appropriate coach and fully dedicate yourself to eliminating chronic pain from your existence. Review your life, study your prior successes and extract their key elements.

If you're so despondent that you cannot uncover any personal strength to support you, read *The Greatest Miracle In The World* by Og Mandino to develop an understanding and appreciation of your true personal worth in the cosmos. Reprogramming your spirit is possible if you believe in yourself. In addition, you might consider a self-help tape series, many of which are readily available. I have personally replaced the taped music collection in my car with the Anthony Robbins *Personal Power* series.

Wake up tomorrow and breathe the air of a new dawn. Start fresh and take your very best step forward. From this day forth, do not look back. Focus all of your energy on succeeding and your positive attitude will give rise to new direction, renewed spirit, unyielding courage and the wonderful feeling of hope that you thought was forgotten or lost.

Step #7
Become An Informed Consumer

Seeking an approach to learning how to help yourself rather than wishing for the instant cure is the major thrust of Step 7. Let's take this opportunity to find a rational chronic pain program, into which you will pour your undivided energies. In Chapter 8, we reviewed the important elements that produce a synergistic effect. You've learned what to expect from a physician and you clearly understand your role in this process. Use your new knowledge to become an informed and effective consumer.

Now is the time to begin your search. You might start by asking your family doctor about a coordinated chronic pain management program. You may consider contacting national pain agencies. The American Association for the Study of Headache, AASH, in New Jersey or The National Headache Foundation in Chicago can be called for recommendations if you suffer from chronic headaches. For other forms of chronic pain, consider contacting the American Academy of Pain Management in California. This organization promotes the multidisciplinary approach and maintains a national registry of pain practitioners. Another reasonable avenue is to call or write the Feldenkrais Guild in Oregon and specifically ask for practitioners in your area who incorporate this form of training into a collaborative pain approach. The addresses and phone numbers of these agencies are listed at the end of this chapter.

Ideally, you will find a practice located near your home. However, if you do have to travel a few hours, consider the fact that the benefits may outweigh the time lost in transit. Some of our patients are willing to travel four or five hours, a few times per week for this type of specialized care. Do not allow the thought of insufficient time to enter your mind, as no more important application of your energies could ever exist. The actual travel experience can provide a wonderful period of solitude that can be utilized to fortify your commitment and review your progress.

On the other hand, do not consider a pain center at a location requiring a trip of sufficient magnitude to impede returning more than a few times per year. This approach is less likely to succeed. You will certainly need close contact and continuity of care.

Researching the location of the pain management center is only the first step. Contact potential choices by phone and thoroughly discuss your questions with a nurse or administrator. Consider calling more than one center and do not proceed if you are not initially satisfied with the center's responses.

In addition, most centers will arrange a consultation with a physician/team leader prior to formally entering a program. Before embarking on this route, study the questions presented at the end of Chapter 8, which provide guidelines for the initial phone contact and the consultation. If the visit with the doctor did not end on a hopeful note or if you are uncomfortable with the approach, reconsider your feelings or discuss them with a loved-one prior to entering the program. Remember, you are an informed consumer with a specific mission to become pain-free. Apply your knowledge and understanding in a logical fashion to seek the very best care possible!

Step #8
Follow Through To Hit The Target

Whether it be tennis, baseball or any similar sport, we have been taught that just initiating the swing is never enough; the follow-through is the key to success. In a similar fashion, beginning a pain program represents only the formal initiation of your commitment. Success can be yours, if you follow through.

One of our most important sources of motivation is the anticipation of a positive change or improvement. In the field of chronic pain management, however, this stimulus does not initially surface. No drug or therapeutic approach can produce an immediate change. You must, therefore, develop the fortitude within yourself to persevere, as improvements will occur slowly and deliberately at first. I often warn my patients that significant changes in their pain profiles will not occur for at least three or four weeks. Improper expectations can falsely lead to the perception of failure, resulting in premature quitting. The physician and team must provide a reasonable timetable for the program and you should understand that unrealistic expectations of immediate success will only worsen your overall syndrome.

Patience is more than a virtue for the chronic pain sufferer; it is a necessity. Don't set goals for yourself that are impractical, as you will certainly sabotage your efforts by developing expectations that cannot be met. Be flexible and accept the possibility of changes within your program, which will often be necessary to assure continued progress. Enjoy your therapy and savor every moment of the learning process. Remember, every day you are getting closer to your goal.

Following through with a chronic pain program is a commitment that will encompass every aspect of your existence. You will most likely be expected to perform routine daily exercises, practice relaxation and biofeedback, follow a diet and decrease or stop using tobacco and alcohol. In addition, precise regulation of medicines is necessary and close contact with the staff will be established. Changes in your daily activities at home or work must parallel your efforts and progress attained within the coordinated therapeutic approach. In effect, you must reprogram your entire self to live a pain-free existence.

The most important advice I can share with you is to become an ACTIVE participant your program. Never forget that progress will unfold through your efforts. Do not expect the cure to happen to you. Success requires your commitment and dedication.

Step #9
Replace Your Pain With Success

The process of freeing yourself from the clutches of chronic pain is multifaceted, requiring a host of endeavors on many levels. Over the years, I have found that my patients are much more likely to succeed if they simultaneously work toward other important goals in their lives. Step 9 is aimed at developing a heightened sense of personal worth through the process of attaining that which has eluded you throughout your life.

For example, if you've always wished to complete your education, set forth this very moment to devise a realistic plan to attain your degree. If you wished to open your own business, seek the advice of experts and develop a logical business strategy. If your goal is to establish a certain relationship, extend yourself to that person.

Deep down inside, you may have arrived at the realization that your true dreams in life were never transformed into reality or, for that matter, ever possible. Such beliefs can serve as catalysts for the evolution of nonproductive programmed responses. The subsequent development of a chronic pain syndrome is no exception.

True happiness must be achieved on many levels. When we're down and out or trapped by a disorder such as chronic pain, our efforts are least likely to be directed toward a lifelong goal. However, as we improve and pain no longer over-shadows our existence, an old and eerie emptiness sometimes surfaces when we face the fact that quality living requires more than just a pain-free existence. After all, living without pain is not a guarantee for happiness or fulfillment. Of concern is the fact that when pain finally diminishes or is eliminated, a true loss is often felt and misinterpreted as painful.

Let's not allow this to happen. Realize that your potential in life extends to more than just conquering pain and develop an effective strategy for attaining a goal that is important to you. Replace the pain in your life with personal success. Do not wait until you are pain-free to approach this issue, as the void that eventually develops may undermine your best efforts. The growth you are now experiencing must occur on many levels simultaneously.

Use your positive attitude and new organizational skills to accomplish goals that are important to you. Your chances of overall success are better than you could ever imagine. The reestablishment of self-respect and harmony will transcend the walls that you have created around you. Your potential is truly unlimited!

205

Step #10
Prevent The Reemergence
of Non-Productive Behaviors

The maintenance of success requires commitment and never-ending energy. The more a musician practices a piece correctly, the more natural, automatic and perfect is the performance. Failure to practice, however, results in reversion to imperfection.

As a physician, I feel rewarded when my patients come back a year after completing our program and state that they feel better than ever. Further improvement in pain management appears to parallel successes in other areas. Unfortunately, a pain-free existence is not easy to maintain for some individuals, for old habits have a tendency to re-emerge.

Sometimes, a person who has successfully completed our program and who has been totally without pain for several months begins to reexperience former symptoms. This is not surprising, in that success is sometimes taken for granted and pain predictably emerges as one slacks off with regard to exercise, diet, relaxation and medication recommendations. Some individuals seem to lose interest in health maintenance, while others attempt to test the waters by straying away from a previously successful program.

Generally, a follow-up visit to review these issues, coupled with a dose of reassurance, is typically all that is needed to reestablish the sure footing that is conducive to maintaining a pain-free existence. For others, regularly scheduled follow-ups, coupled with specialized programs for personal development are necessary.

The key to Step 10 is not allowing your old patterns of thinking or action, which originally fostered your suffering, to reemerge. In order to maintain a pain-free state, you must remain constantly vigilant. Those old habits, doubts and weaknesses must be reprogrammed into health-maintaining activities, confidence, drive and strength. Having once achieved a state of success, you owe it to yourself to sustain it. A positive outlook, coupled with unrelenting faith, hope and fortitude will assure prosperity for the rest of your life.

Conclusions

The intimate relationship between mind and body is truly inseparable. Our knowledge and understanding dictates that reasonable approaches for chronic pain sufferers must address this union. *Reprogramming Pain* is more than just an all-encompassing review of this problem. It is a practical "how to" manual, written to help you recognize the learned responses that trigger and perpetuate your suffering. Ten important steps have been presented to form the foundation for an effective strategy to reprogram your life. Let's take a moment to review them.

Ten Steps For Reprogramming Pain

1. Take action.
2. Perform a "Personal Reflections" Inventory.
3. Study your pain and movement patterns.
4. Survey your external influences.
5. Face ongoing conflicts.
6. Incorporate personal strengths into a positive attitude.
7. Become an informed consumer.
8. Follow through to hit the target.
9. Replace your pain with success.
10. Prevent the reemergence of nonproductive behaviors.

As a human being, you are more than just the expression of a genetic code of DNA helices. You are the product of experience, associations and societal programming, which condition your behavioral responses in ways that are often detrimental to your health. Despite your individual character, you predictably respond to a variety of influences that mold and shape even your deepest feelings.

Ultimately, you alone have the power to shape your destiny. Your decision to live without chronic pain must represent the conscious effort of your entire being. You must enlist all of your energy to develop a positive approach and combine it with an unyielding desire to improve the quality of your existence. Your limits are determined only by your imagination.

Richard Bach, in his world renowned classic, *Jonathan Livingston Seagull*, addresses this very issue. In a conversation with a seagull named Fletcher, Jonathan exclaims:

> Don't believe what your eyes are telling
> you. All they show is limitation. Look
> with your understanding, find out what
> you already know, and you'll see the
> way to fly.

Opening your mind to reestablish faith in yourself will build your strength. Dedicate yourself to developing an improved awareness of your mind and body and never forget their unity. Cast aside your personal doubts, while initiating a new and wonderful course to success. Invest in your own well-being and begin the process of ...

REPROGRAMMING PAIN!

For Additional Information

call or write:

**Headache Center Neurology Institute
of Western Pennsylvania**
P.O. Box 1388
Meadville, PA 16335
Phone: (814) 724-1765

American Academy of Pain Management
3600 Sisk Road Suite 2D
Modesto, CA 95356
Phone: (209) 545-0754

**The American Association for the
Study of Headache**
875 Kings Highway, Suite 200
Woodbury, NJ 08096
Phone: (800) 255-2243

National Headache Foundation
5252 North Western Avenue
Chicago, IL 60625
Phone: (800) 843-2256

The Feldenkrais Guild
524 Ellsworth Street
P.O. Box 489
Albany, OR 97321-0143
Phone: (503) 926-0981

Recommended Reading

Bach, R. (1970). <u>Jonathan Livingston Seagull</u>. New York: Avon.

Benson, H. and Klipper, M.Z. (1975). <u>The Relaxation Response</u>. New York: Avon.

Benson, H. and Proctor, W. (1984). <u>Beyond the Relaxation Response</u>. New York: Berkley.

Borysenko, J. (1987). <u>Minding The Body, Mending The Mind</u>. New York: Bantam.

Chopra, D. (1993). <u>Ageless Body, Timeless Mind</u>. New York: Harmony.

Cousins, N. (1989). <u>Head First</u>. New York: Penguin.

Dossey, L. (1993). <u>Healing Words</u>. New York: HarperCollins.

Dyer, W. (1992). <u>Real Magic</u>. New York: HarperCollins.

Feldenkrais, M. (1984). <u>The Master Moves</u>. Cupertino, CA: Meta.

Hanna, T. (1 988). <u>Somatics</u>. Reading, MA: Addison-Wesley.

Mandino, 0. (1977). <u>The Greatest Miracle in the World</u>. New York: Bantam.

Moyers, B. (1993). <u>Healing and The Mind</u>. New York: Bantam.

Pulos, L. (1990). <u>Beyond Hypnosis</u>. San Francisco: Omega.

Pulos, L. and Richman, G. (1990). <u>Miracles and Other Realities</u>. San Francisco: Omega.

Siegel, B.S. (1993). <u>How To Live Between Office Visits</u>. New York: HarperCollins.

Siegel, B.S. (1989). <u>Peace Love & Healing</u>, New York: Harper & Row.

Index

A

AASH, 201
Activities, 101 – 106
Acupuncture, 33
ADHD, 140
Advertising campaigns, 39, 77 – 79, 80
Alarm, personal systems, 123
Alcohol, 114 – 117, 154, 171
Alexander, Frederick M., 65
Allen, James, 167, 199
American Academy of Pain Management, 201
American Association for Study of Headache, 201
Anxiety, 123, 128
Anxiolytics, 150
Appearances, 38
Approaches,
    medical, 153 – 155
    psychological, 157 – 158
    physical, 155 – 157
    relaxation, 100
    traditional, 148 – 152
Arthritis, 67
Association areas, 29
Associations, 39
    banging it back, 83
    painful, 39
    past, 80 – 82
    pleasurable, 39
    programmed, 80
Athletes, 56
Attention deficit disorders, 128
Attitude, positive, 199 – 200
Autonomic nervous system, 34 – 35, 125, 130, 133

Awareness Through Movement, 62 – 65, 156

B

Bach, Richard, 209
Bedside manner, 116
Behavior,
    non–productive, 206 – 207
    pain, 30 – 33
benShea, Noah, 186
Benson, M.D., Herbert, 180, 181
Berk, Dr.P.H., Lee, 36, 175
Biofeedback, 49, 100, 126 – 129, 135 – 137, 147, 158
Borysenko, Ph.D., Joan, 131
Brain, 22 – 27
Brodmann's areas, 26
Building Fear, 186
Bulging disc, 44

C

Caffeinated beverages, 113 – 114
Central processing unit, 25
Chopra, M.D., Deepak, 180
Circuitry, protective, 21 – 22, 30
Coach, 144
Computer, the brain as, 22 – 27
Conclusions, scientific, 174 – 176
Concussion, 48
Conditioning, 138
Conflicts, ongoing 197 – 198
Consumer, informed 200 – 202
Control 123
Convergent therapy 152, 157 – 160, 163, 171
Cortex, somatosensory, 26
Cousins, Norman, 145, 182

215

CPU, 25
Cringing, 71
CT scans, 166
Cure, instant, 16, 82 – 84, 118
Cure me attitude, 144

D

Dan's Story, 48 – 50
David's Story, 12 – 16
Deborah's Story, 2 – 5
Deception, sensory, 70
Development, human,
   experiences, 38
   learning processes, 38
Diet, 112 – 114, 154
Disc bulging, 44, 45, 46
Doctor, 116 – 119
Doctor shopping, 14
Dorsal Raphe Nucleus, 31
Dossey, M.D., Larry, 182
Double–blinded studies, 174
Dyer, M.D., Wayne, 182

E

EEG, 48
Emotions,
   factors, 41
   overlay, 40
   programming, 88 – 90
Endorphins, 33
Expression, muscular, 63

F

Factor, triggering, 133, 134
Fads, 78
Fashion, 18
Fear, 187
Feldenkrais, Moshe, 62,
     63, 67, 68, 156
Feldenkrais Guild, 201

Fibromyalgia, 45
Fight or flight response, 34
Follow–through, 202 – 204
Force, higher, 179 – 183
Frustration, 106 – 108

G

Gate Theory, 32
Gelb, Michael, 65
Gibran, Kahlil, 172
Groups, research,
   control, 174 – 175
   experimental, 174

H

Hanna, Ph.D., Thomas, 69, 168
Harvard Medical School, 131
Headache, 47, 94
   aura 129
   drug rebound, 86, 87
   transformed migraine, 87
   tension, 40
Healer image, 144
Health, 176
Henderson, Reverend Charles, 186
Hip fracture, 66
Homunculus, 27
Hypnosis, 49
Hypnotherapists, 147

I

Imagery, 131
Images, 91 – 92
Inactivity, 61
Influences, external, 194 – 197
Inhibition, programmed, 71
Injury, 2, 11
Invisible navigator, 37, 50, 53

J

Jason's Story, 51–52
Jennifer's Story, 43–47

L

Laughter, 36
Listening to your body, 56–61

M

Mandino, Og, 177–178, 183, 200
Manipulations, 100
Map, body, 191
Margolis, M.D., Michael, 113
Marquis, Donald Robert Perry, 169
Massage, 100
Massage therapists, 147
Media industry, 76
Medical director, 159
Medication,
    NSAIDS, 85
    off–the–shelf, 84
    over–the–counter, 50, 85, 91, 98
    potential pitfalls, 86
    prescription, 98–99
Melzak and Wall, 32
Mind/body balance, 122
Mindscope®, 129, 137–141
Movement, patterns of, 61, 190–194
Moyers, Bill, 175
MRI scans, 166

N

National Headache Foundation,
    84, 201
Nerve, 44, 45
    pinched, 44, 45
Nervous system,
    autonomic, 34–35
    central, 22, 25–27

peripheral, 22–23
Neuropeptide, 33
Neurosis, 40
Neurotransmitters, 24, 31
Nielsen Media Research, 76
NSAIDs, 85
Numbness, 44
Nutrition, 112

O

Ornish, M.D., Dean, 181, 182
Over–the–counter, 84–85, 91, 98

P

Pain,
    behavior, 30–33, 75
    circuitry, 35
    definition of, 7–8
    medication, 85–88
    practitioners, 147
    receptors, 22
    words associated with, 42
Panic disorders, 128
Patients, professional, 149
Personal fitness trainers, 147
Personal Power, 200
Personal Reflections Inventory,
    95, 101, 119, 121, 188–190
Pert, Ph.D., Candace, 34, 175, 176
Physical therapist, 151
Physical therapy, 100, 157
Physician–patient relationship, 118,
    144–147
Pinched nerve, 44
Placebo, 174, 175
PMS premenstrual syndrome, 31
Postures, defensive, 71
Primitive reflex response, 28
Processing, 25
Procrastination, 169

217

Programming
  emotions, 88
  images, 91
  trust, 90
Programs, multidisciplinary, 160
PRN, 111
The Prophet, 172
Processes, psychological, 157
Psychoneuroimmunology, 35, 36
Psychosomatic, 41, 134, 174
Pulos, Ph.D., Lee, 131, 182, 184

Q
Quick fix, 171
Quitting, 169

R
Rebound, drug, 87
Receptors, 28
Reflections, Personal, 94 – 96
Reflex, primitive, 28
Reflex Sympathetic Dystrophy, 128 – 129
  definition of, 35
Relaxation Response, 180
Reprogramming Pain Inventory, 42, 195
Responses, 28, 61
  central nervous system, 51
  fight or flight, 34
  flexion and tightening, 71
  improper psychological, 61
  primitive reflex, 28
  programmed, 129 – 135
Richman, Gary, 184
Robbins, Anthony, 78 – 80, 200
Runner's high, 33

S
Sadie's Story, 66 – 69

Self–worth, 105
Sensory deception, 69 – 71
Siegel, M.D., Bernie, 145, 162, 182
Skating, 70 – 73
Skiing, 57 – 58
Smoking, 114 – 116, 154, 171
Spasm, 61
Spirit, human, 166 – 173
Splinting, 60
Stereotypes, 83
Strength, personal, 199 – 200
Stress, 7, 123
Substances, illicit, 154
Substance P, 33
Success, 183 – 184, 204 – 205
Suffering, 8
Susan's Story, 9 – 12
Synapses, 24, 30
  excitatory, 32
  inhibitory, 32
Synergy, 5, 143, 153, 158 – 162

T
Taking Action, 186 – 187
Television, 76 – 78
Ten Steps, 185 – 207
TENS, 32, 33, 156
Tobacco, 114 – 116, 171
Trust, 90

V
Vitamins, 113, 115

W
Wickram, Ph.D., Ian, 124
Words (associated with pain), 42
Work, 96 – 97

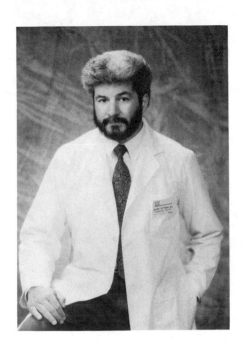

About The Author

Barry B. Bittman, M.D., neurologist, is the director of the Headache Center Neurology Institute of western Pennsylvania. Dr. Bittman is the author of several medical articles in the field of pain management and computer applications in rehabilitation. He serves on the editorial boards of the Journal of Neurological and Orthopedic Medicine and Surgery and the American Journal of Pain Management. Dr. Bittman's most recent focus is centered on his invention, MINDSCOPE®, the first mind guided interactive multimedia system in the world. He and his wife, Karen have three children, Benjamin, Marcus and Lauren.